Medicolegal Essentials in Healthcare

2nd Edition

D0898649

Medicolegal Essentials in Healthcare

2nd Edition

Edited by

Jason Payne-James LLM FRCS DFM RNutr
Forensic Physician, London
Principal Forensic Physician,
City of London Police, and
Director, Forensic Healthcare Services Ltd

Ian Wall LLM DCH DRCOG MRCGP
Barister at Law, and
Forensic Physician
London

Peter Dean MBBS BDS (Hons) DRCOG LLM
H.M. Coroner
Greater Suffolk and South East Essex, and
Forensic Medical Examiner
London

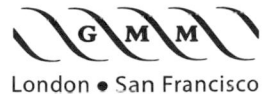
London • San Francisco

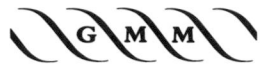

© 2004

Greenwich Medical Media Limited
137 Euston Road
London NW1 2AA

870 Market Street, Ste 720,
San Francisco, CA 94102

ISBN 184110 1702

First published 1996
Second edition published 2004

A catalogue record for this book is available from the British Library.

Typeset by Charon Tec Pvt. Ltd, Chennai, India

Printed in the UK by The Alden Group, Oxford

Visit our website at **www.greenwich-medical.co.uk**

Contents

Contributors

Hazel Biggs BA PhD
Senior Lecturer and Director of Medical Law
University of Kent
Canterbury, Kent, UK

Peter Dean MB BS BDS (Hons) DRCOG LLM
H.M. Coroner
Greater Suffolk and South East Essex and
Forensic Medical Examiner
London, UK

George Fernie LLB MB ChB MPhil MRCGP DFM
Medico-Legal Adviser
Medical and Dental Defence Union of Scotland and
Honorary Senior Lecturer
Department of Forensic Medicine
University of Glasgow, UK

Alain Gregoire MBBS DRCOG MRCPsych
Consultant Psychiatrist
Perinatal Mental Health Service
Southampton, UK

Robin Harman PhD MRPharmS
Independent Pharmaceutical and Regulatory Consultant
Farnham, Surrey, UK

Sharon Korek BSc LLB LLM JP
Senior Lecturer in Law
University of Hertfordshire, UK

Allan Levy Q.C.
Barrister at Law, London, and
Senior Visiting Fellow
Southampton University Law School, UK

Adrian Lower FRCOG
Consultant Gynaecologist, and
Medical Director
Isis Fertility Centre
Colchester, UK

Felicity Nicholson BSc FRCPath
Forensic Physician, and
Consultant Specialist in Infectious Diseases
London, UK

Jason Payne-James LLM FRCS DFM RNutr
Forensic Physician, London
Principal Forensic Physician
City of London Police, and
Director, Forensic Healthcare Services Ltd, UK

Michael Peel MB BS MRCGP MFOM DMJ
Health and Human Rights Adviser
Medical Foundation for the Care of Victims of Torture
London, UK

Steve Robinson MB ChB DMJ
Senior Police Surgeon
Greater Manchester Police, and
Honorary Lecturer in Forensic Medicine
University of Manchester, UK

Christobel Saunders MB BS FRCS FRCS (Gen) FRACS
Professor of Surgical Oncology
School of Surgery & Pathology
University of Western Australia, Australia

Peter Schütte MB ChB DipMRCGP DMJ (Clin) DA DRCOG
Acting Head of Advisory Services
Medical Defence Union
London, UK

Julie Smith BA PhD
Honorary Fellow of Bristol University
Department of Paediatric Epidemiology, and
Non-Executive Director
Southend Hospital NHS Trust, UK

Sue Sutherland RGN RM DPM
Chief Executive
UK Transplant
Bristol, UK

Ian Wall LLM DCH, DRCOG MRCGP
Barrister at Law, and
Forensic Physician
London, UK

Michael Wilks MB BS DRCOG
Principal Forensic Medical Examiner
Metropolitan Police, London,
Chairman, Medical Ethics Committee
British Medical Association
London, UK

Editors' note for the first edition

The aim of this book is to provide an overview of those legal issues most relevant to individuals working in the healthcare professions. The need for a basic understanding of the legal framework in which healthcare is provided, and of the role that law and the judiciary play in the working lives of all such professionals, is now being recognised and by the increasing emphasis placed on the teaching of legal and ethical principles to undergraduate students in medicine, nursing, pharmacy and allied professions. Knowledge of these subjects has become an intrinsic part of many teaching courses, and there is no part of the wide spectrum of healthcare provision that does not, at some time, require an understanding and consideration of these basic medicolegal principles. Those professionals already qualified and in practice, both in hospitals and the community, regularly experience the need to have appropriate knowledge of many of these issues. With increasing frequency items of medicolegal significance appear in the news and media. This book looks at those areas where law and medicine commonly meet. The chapters are written by a multidisciplinary group of practitioners with special interest or experience in their subjects. We hope that these medicolegal essentials will provide a sound basis for undergraduates, postgraduates and all healthcare providers, and will inspire some to develop, further their own interest, knowledge and understanding of the growing and increasingly important interface between medicine and the law.

The law in this book is stated as of April 1 1996.

JP-J, PD, IW   London 1996

Editors' note for the second edition

Since the publication of the first edition of Medicolegal Essentials in Healthcare, the need for all healthcare professionals to be aware of and have a basic understanding of the legal issues that confront us on a daily basis has, if anything, increased. The provision of healthcare is being scrutinised in a way that would have been unimaginable even two decades ago. In the UK barely a day goes by without a significant medicolegal issue being debated in the media. Recent years have seen inquiries and reports with which names such as Bristol, Alder Hey, Shipman, and Climbie have become synonymous – each of which has addressed issues crucial to healthcare and which, in part, may reflect the limited extent of the training provided in legal and ethical issues for most working in this area. As medical technology and skills increase, so it seems that issues that some perceive as peripheral concerning the legal framework in which we practice are neglected in undergraduate training. It is our belief that a basic knowledge of the medicolegal issues of healthcare is a prerequisite for safe, responsible and ethical practice – whatever our field of work. This book refers to the legal and healthcare system in England and Wales, but broad principles may be applied across many jurisdictions. We hope that this book goes some way towards providing the core information relating to good medicolegal practice of which we need to be aware.

JP-J
IW
PD
London 2004

Note
The law in this book is stated as of 1st November 2003.
The contents of this book follow the Interpretation Act 1978, so in that unless specifically stated otherwise, words importing the masculine gender include the feminine and words importing the feminine gender include the masculine.

Foreword

In recent years there has been a cultural shift in the perceptions surrounding professional relationships in the area of healthcare. The widespread dissemination of specialist medical information has encouraged patients to adopt a more consumerist role, to question their treatment, and to seek explanations when expected standards are not realised. The provision of medical care has also undergone considerable changes. Means of diagnosis and treatment have multiplied with technological advances, but this has often resulted in an uncomfortable game of catch-up between expectations and outcome. Technology has resulted in the ability of doctors to manipulate life and death and to challenge fundamental notions of the human condition. The focus of medical practice is often on rules of science, and this book looks at medicine from the wider context where rules of custom and law are also important considerations. A vast number of important subject are covered; from controversial issues such as euthanasia, living wills, organ donation and reproductive health, to issues such as consent and confidentiality, which form the very foundation of the doctor/patient relationship. The second edition of this book provides a comprehensive collection of chapters on medicolegal issues, and should be in the bookcase of every health professional, and perhaps every lawyer.

Dame Elizabeth Butler-Sloss, DBE
President of the Family Division
Royal Courts of Justice

March 2004

Table of statutes

Table of cases

1

Legal institutions and the legal process

Ian Wall and Jason Payne-James

Few areas of healthcare practice are untouched by the law, and health care professionals will no doubt have some involvement with the legal process during their careers. This chapter seeks to provide an overview of the salient and relevant features of the legal system in England and Wales, in order to facilitate an understanding of the subject matter in the subsequent chapters.

Scotland and Northern Ireland enjoy their own legal traditions which, though distinct from that of England and Wales, share many similarities.

SOURCES OF LAW

Laws are rules that govern orderly behaviour in a collective society. The system which we call 'the Law', is an expression of the formal institutionalisation of the promulgation, adjudication, and enforcement of rules.

In England and Wales, the principal sources of these laws are Parliament and the decisions of judges in courts of law. Increasingly, however, rule-making powers are now the subject of delegation.

Parliamentary law

Parliament is the principal and pre-eminent organ of legislation in the UK. It is composed of the House of Commons, the House of Lords and the Monarch. In theory, the political and legal doctrine of 'Parliamentary Sovereignty', means that Parliament can pass any law it sees fit, and such laws cannot be altered by the courts.

In order to achieve the status of an Act of Parliament, the proposed Parliamentary legislation (known as a 'Bill') must successfully negotiate a series of 'readings' in both Houses, as well as a detailed scrutiny of its provisions by a 'Standing Committee'.

Delegated legislation

Parliament has neither the time nor the flexibility to produce Statutes that might anticipate every individual detail of its subject matter.

Statutes, therefore, often contain broad permissive provisions delegating legislative powers to government ministers as well as a plethora of 'public bodies' associated with government departments.

The legislative product of such properly delegated power, (known variously as statutory instruments (SIs), 'bye-laws', rules and regulations), possess the same force of law as the parent or enabling Act of Parliament.

Government ministers and their departments are responsible for issuing some 3000 SIs annually, as well as the myriad of circulars, codes and 'guidances' emanating from the state, the resulting figure represents a significant legislative power when compared to the 50 or so statutes passed annually.

Ministers and government departments receive administrative assistance in the detailed execution of policy from over one thousand 'independent' public bodies known as Non Departmental Public Bodies (NDPBs). NDPBs cast a wide shadow into all areas of public activity and they themselves are often sub-delegated the responsibility to formulate rules and regulations. While this method of legislation has both the advantage of flexibility as well as utilising sources of specialist knowledge, it is both opaque and lacking in public accountability.

STRUCTURE OF THE NATIONAL HEALTH SERVICE

A statutory creation, the National Health Service (NHS), was introduced in 1948 to bring the provision of healthcare under direct government responsibility in order to ensure a free and comprehensive service. Overall responsibility for the NHS currently rests with the Secretary of State for Health who, assisted by a number of Ministers of Health, heads the Department of Health.

The NHS and its institutions are the subject of frequent structural changes, and at present the Department of Health exercises direct control over the Strategic Health Authorities and indirect control over NHS Trusts, Primary Care Trusts, and Care Trusts.

While in theory government ministers are *responsible* for their individual fiefdom, personal ministerial control of this vast organisation is not possible. The administration and implementation of government policy operates, therefore, by way of delegation of discretionary powers through to the various administrative tiers within the service.

Control of executive powers

The NHS is one of the principal organs of the UK's welfare system and as a state emanation has the potential to impinge on individual rights and freedoms, a position aggravated by delegation of the practical implementation of policy to unelected and unaccountable administrative bodies.

There are a variety of political and legal controls, of varying effectiveness, on these state sponsored powers.

Ministerial responsibility

Ministers may be required to answer open questions from the floor in Parliament on both their actions and those of their department. This may often represent a source of considerable political embarrassment, as well as unwelcome media and public attention, though in practice, matters are often disposed of by way of written replies.

Parliamentary review and Select Committees

Parliamentary Select Committees sit to examine expenditure, administration, and policy of government departments and associated public bodies. Members of Parliament from each political persuasion are represented, and individual membership is often a consequence of a special interest in a particular area.

The two Select Committees which are primarily concerned with health matters, the Select Committee on Health, and the Public Administration Select Committee, have wide powers to examine documents and summon persons before them.

Tribunals

Tribunals are 'public' bodies established to deal with conflicts that arise between the citizens and administrative bodies, to ensure that delegated discretionary powers are properly exercised.

There are now some 70 different administrative tribunals in England and Wales, dealing with around one million cases per annum.

Statutory tribunals, such as the Mental Health Review Tribunal[1], are creations of primary legislation, though there exist a number of 'domestic tribunals' established pursuant to agreement between private individuals (e.g. the Jockey Club).

Though primarily 'administrative' in nature, many tribunals operate in a quasi-judicial capacity.

The effectiveness of tribunals as independent checks on executive power is questionable, particularly when most depend on the sponsoring Department of State for administrative support, expenses, and appointment of members.[2]

Tribunals deal with a considerably greater volume of cases than the civil courts. They are reputed to benefit from being flexible, cheap, and to possess relevant specialist expertise, thereby enabling them to deal with cases more expeditiously. Tribunals may be subject to judicial scrutiny by way of judicial review (infra).

Public inquiries

Departments of State often establish *ad hoc* internal private inquiries to examine alleged wrongdoing within their sphere of influence. Where, however, the issues involved are likely to arouse national concern, the relevant Secretary of State can seek a resolution of both Houses of Parliament to establish a statutory public inquiry with formal terms of reference.

These inquiries though having powers to compel witnesses to attend and testify under oath, are not courts of law; they adopt an inquisitorial process and seek primarily to establish truth.

Public inquiries are lengthy and costly affairs and often by the time they report their findings, and make their recommendations, public feeling has moved on.

The Ombudsman

The Office of The Parliamentary Commissioner for Administration (PCA)[3] was created in 1967. A Crown appointee and independent of the government, the PCA (or ombudsman) is charged with the investigation of maladministration on the part of government or government agencies.

The Health Service Ombudsman (HSO) specifically investigates complaints that hardship or injustice has been caused by the NHS's failure to provide a service, or where there has been an administrative failure (maladministration).[4] It is the decision-making *process* that forms the basis of any investigation and not the *merits* of the individual case (see also Chapter 7).

Aggrieved persons (or their family) can access the PCA via their MP, and between 2000 and 2001 the HSO considered 870 cases ranging from waiting times to standards of diagnosis and care. The HSO produces an annual report with appropriate recommendations that is examined by a Select Committee and on which the government is encouraged to act. The HSO will only investigate complaints that have first passed through the local complaints procedures.

The Ombudsman has no powers to examine complaints that could be taken to court, matters relating to government policy, decision *properly* arrived at by NHS bodies, or issues of a 'personal' nature such as contracts of employment.

Judicial review

The High Court maintains an inherent supervisory jurisdiction over inferior courts, tribunals, and administrative bodies exercising delegated judicial and quasi-judicial powers in the public domain. Individuals aggrieved by the actions of these bodies may seek redress through the courts by way of an application for *judicial review.*

The High Court will exercise its 'public law' jurisdiction only where a public body has made an error of law, has acted 'illegally', 'irrationally', or where there has been 'procedural impropriety'. These grounds have been held to include matters such as a body acting outside the powers (*ultra vires*) that have been delegated to it, acting unreasonably, acting with bad faith, or for improper purposes.

In policing the exercise of discretionary powers by public bodies, the High Courts are mindful of balancing the need to protect individual freedoms from undue and oppressive interference by the organs of government, while also ensuring an efficient executive. It is not the role of the courts to usurp the decision-making powers *rightly* delegated by Parliament to public bodies particularly where such delegation is predicated on the greater substantive expertise possessed by many of these bodies in their particular areas of operation.

An application for judicial review requires the leave of the High Court, and will only be granted in cases that raise 'public law' issues, and where the aggrieved party can demonstrate a 'sufficient interest' in the outcome of the case (known as *locus standi*). In this way, the courts can weed out vexatious claims.

The process of judicial review only allows the 'supervising' court to invalidate an illegal decision, and send it back to the original deciding body for reconsideration. Judicial review is concerned with procedural issues and not the substantive issues.[5] The supervising court cannot substitute its own opinion on the substantive merits of the decision, and in this important aspect judicial review differs from appeal.

The limitations of judicial review exposes a lacuna in the legal protection of substantive individual rights; rendered all the more acute by an absence of a written constitution in the UK.

Human Rights Act 1998 (see also Chapter 2)

The Human Rights Act (HRA) has given UK courts greater power to protect certain fundamental rights by introducing the European Convention on Human Rights (and the related jurisprudence) into UK domestic law.

The European Convention seeks to protect certain fundamental rights of its citizens such as the right to life (Article 2), liberty (Article 5), privacy (Article 8), and a family life (Article 12). The HRA has introduced a rights-based 'constitution' into UK domestic law and all legislation must now be compatible with these rights.

In deference to Parliamentary Sovereignty, and the constitutional effects of a notional shift in power to the judiciary, s19 HRA expressly states that the courts cannot invalidate incompatible primary legislation. The courts can nevertheless make a declaration of incompatibility and allow the legislature to remedy it, *should it so desire*. Furthermore, as part of Parliamentary procedure, ministers sponsoring Bills must make a statement of compatibility with Convention rights (s19 HRA).

Subordinate legislation, in contrast, may be struck down by the courts if it cannot be construed as compatible with rights granted under the Convention.

In addition to these legislative checks, s6 HRA makes it illegal for 'public authorities' or persons exercising functions of a public nature to act in any way that is incompatible with Convention rights, unless, under the relevant statutory provisions, the authority could not have acted differently.

The term 'public authority' is not defined, but is intended to be interpreted widely and would certainly include the panoply of administrative bodies associated with the machinery of healthcare provision in the UK.

JUDICIAL LAW

The other principal source of law in the UK arises from the corpus of decisions made by judges in the courts. This form of law has evolved over time and is often referred to as 'common law' or 'case law'. It was, until the 17th century, the pre-eminent source of law in the UK, and while Statute Law has since superseded it in terms of sheer bulk, case law still enjoys an important role.

Consistency and fairness in judicial law is maintained to a certain extent by the 'doctrine of precedent' which ensures that the principles enunciated in one court will normally be binding on judges in inferior courts in subsequent cases. The House of Lords, by way of exception, is not so bound, and has jurisdiction to overrule its previous decisions.

Allied to the concept of Parliamentary Sovereignty is that of a judiciary that is independent of state control, though the provisions of statutory law will always bind the courts. The courts have always exercised a role in construing or interpreting statutory language, but with the introduction of the HRA the courts may now enjoy greater powers.

Branches of law

The law is divided into a number of specialist fields, each with its own language, procedures and substantive rules; the two principal categories being civil law and criminal law.

Civil law is concerned with the resolution of disputes between individuals. It is the aggrieved party who undertakes the legal action (a 'suit') and remedies are usually financial.

Criminal law is concerned with the relationship between individuals and the state. Where the nature of an act is of sufficient importance or gravity, the state will undertake the 'prosecution' of an individual, and the sentences are punitive in nature.

There is an overlap between these two jurisdictions and a criminal offence (e.g. assault) will often have an equivalent in the civil jurisdiction (e.g. trespass).

As a reflection of this division, the courts are similarly split into civil and criminal jurisdiction with each jurisdiction being arranged in a hierarchical manner reflecting precedent and expertise.

In both jurisdictions the conduct of the litigation is adversarial in nature.

The Civil Courts in England and Wales

The Magistrates' Court is the lowest of the civil courts in England and Wales, and, outside family, and matrimonial issues, has a limited role in civil disputes. 'Lay' magistrates sit in the majority of Magistrate Courts and are advised by a legally qualified justices' clerk. In metropolitan areas, however, a legally qualified District Judge (Magistrate Court) will sit alone.

Above the Magistrates' Court is the County Court, where, in the presence of a circuit judge, 90% of all civil disputes are heard annually.

The High Court has unlimited jurisdiction in civil cases, and hears cases which involve more complex legal issues and/or cases involving high monetary values.

The High Court itself comprises of three divisions: the Chancery Division, which specialises in matters such as company law and trusts; the Family Division, specialising in matrimonial issues and matters relating to minors; and the Queen's Bench Division, which deals with general civil matters. It is usual for judges in the High Court to sit in the absence of a jury.

The High Court sits in the Royal Courts of Justice in London, but has a number of provincial offices known as district registries.

The Divisional Court of the Queen's Bench is a distinct entity that exercises its jurisdiction in respect of certain appeals from Magistrates' Courts (on civil matters), tribunals, and judicial review.

The Civil Division of the Court of Appeal will hear appeals on matters of law (and are therefore not retrials) from the High Court and the County Courts, and is presided over by the Master of the Rolls and the Lords Justices of Appeal.

The ultimate appellate civil court for England and Wales, Scotland, and Northern Ireland is the House of Lords sitting in a judicial capacity.

The Judicial Committee of the Privy Council

This court is composed of 'Councillors' who have occupied senior judicial positions. It has a domestic appellate jurisdiction in respect of decisions of disciplinary committees of the General Medical Council and other statutory healthcare related bodies, as well as a civil and criminal appellate jurisdiction in respect of certain Commonwealth countries.

The Criminal Courts in England and Wales

The Magistrates' Courts play an important role in the criminal jurisdiction, hearing the vast majority of minor criminal cases.

The Crown Court is a single court that sits in a number of different 'tiered' centres throughout England and Wales. It is the court of first instance in respect of the more serious, or 'indictable', offences, but also hears appeals from Magistrates Courts on points of law or against conviction and/or sentence.

Appeals from the Crown Court are made to the Criminal division of the Court of Appeal, presided over by the Lord Chief Justice and the Vice President of the Criminal Division, and thence to the House of Lords on important points of law.

Individuals under the age of 18 will be tried at special Youth Courts.

Coroner Courts

These are ancient courts in English law and unique in respect of their inquisitorial approach. The coroners jurisdiction is over certain categories of death, and inquests are held to determine the 'how, where and when' of a death, and not to apportion blame or to opine on criminal or civil liability (see Chapter 9).

REFERENCES

1. Mental Health Act 1985.
2. See Human Rights Act 1998 and Article 6 European Convention on Human Rights; and Right to a Fair Hearing.
3. The Parliamentary Commissioner Act 1967 (www.parliament.ombudsman.org.uk).
4. www.ombudsman.org.uk
5. See *supra* HSO.

See generally

A. The English Legal System (5th Edition), Gary Slapper and David Kelly, Cavendish Publishing Limited, 2001.
B. Human Rights; The 1998 Act and the European Convention. Stephen Grosz, Jack Beatson, Peter Duffy, Sweet and Maxwell, 2000.
C. Judicial Review and Crown Office Practice, Richard Gordon, Sweet and Maxwell, 1999.

2

Human rights and healthcare professionals

Michael Peel

HUMAN RIGHTS

The concept of human rights is that people have inherent rights simply because they are human. The ideas that developed during the Renaissance were that all men (but not generally at that stage, women or children) were equal. This was either for religious reasons, such as the Protestant view that as all men were created in God's image they must be equal, or because it was a fundamental principle in their secular humanist philosophy. They should therefore, be treated equally by the law. They, or according to many political philosophers, those with some degree of social standing, have the right to try to influence political decisions that affect them. Their personal lives and possessions should not be interfered with arbitrarily. These formulations are equivalent to the biomedical ethics, principles of justice, autonomy and non-maleficence respectively (see also Chapter 3).

It is possible to find references to some of the concepts that later became those of human rights in such documents as the Code of Hammurabi (1780 BCE) and Aristotle's Nichomachean Ethics (330 BCE). One of the first legal instruments in the UK covering human rights issues was the Magna Carta (1215), in articles such as:

> (39). No freeman shall be seized, or imprisoned, or dispossessed, or outlawed, or in any way destroyed; nor will we condemn him, nor will we commit him to prison, excepting by the legal judgement of his peers, or by the laws of the land.

Up to this point the King's word was law (the Divine Right of Kings) so justice was, at best, arbitrary. Subsequently, men of property gained some rights against the absolute rule of the king. However, more than 400 years later the balance between human rights and the Divine Right of Kings was still being debated at the time of the English Civil Wars (1642–1651). The philosophical arguments were developed in books by authors such as John Locke (e.g. Two Treatises of Government, 1680) and Jean-Jacques Rousseau (e.g. The Social Contract, 1762), which were in turn influential on the American Declaration of Independence (1776) and the French Declaration of the Rights of Man and the Citizen (1789).[1] However, the concept of human rights was criticised by many. Jeremy Bentham, for example, described human rights in general and the French Declaration in particular as 'nonsense on stilts' because, amongst other reasons, he considered that rights were meaningless unless they were enforceable. (Anarchical Fallacies; Being an Examination of the Declarations of Rights Issued during the French Revolution, 1823.)[2]

The next stage in the process came after the horrors of the Second World War. More than 30 rights were listed in the Universal Declaration of Human Rights (UDHR, 1948),[3] which was adopted by the General Assembly of the UN and is now accepted by all Member States as a precondition of entry to the UN. Eighteen years later, they were effectively split into two groups. The International Covenant on Economic, Social and Cultural Rights (ICESCR, 1966) includes the rights to work, education, health and social security. The International Covenant on Civil and Political Rights (ICCPR, 1966) includes the rights to life, liberty and a fair trial, and freedom from torture and slavery. Specific UN conventions have been agreed on a range of issues, including genocide,[4] torture,[5] discrimination against women,[6] and on the rights of the child.[7] There has also been some work on prosecuting perpetrators of gross human rights abuses.[8] However, generally breaches of these covenants and conventions are not legally enforceable other than in parallel structures such as the International Criminal Tribunals for Rwanda and for the former Yugoslavia. Mostly they rely on a system of 'naming and shaming' that is rarely publicised in national media, although many countries go to considerable lengths to avoid their breaches being publicised.

Human rights appertain to the individual and put limits on what a state can do to that person. They are independent of the state, so even in a democratic state, there cannot be a vote to take away anyone's human rights. Some rights are absolute, such as the right not to be held in slavery. Some are qualified, such as the right to liberty, which permits detention following certain legitimate procedures. Others, mostly social, economic and cultural rights, require a state to strive to achieve them. As a consequence of a person having a right, there will be a duty on another person or institution (an agent). A right can entail a 'negative' duty, such as not torturing the person, or a 'positive' duty such as providing basic education. Only states are subject to international human rights law. They bind a state, and as a part of that positive obligation the right entails to protect the rights listed, so there are obligations on states for both 'negative' and 'positive' rights. In the case of the right to life, for example, this will mean that the state has a positive duty to criminalize murder. The state must pass appropriate legislation, inform people of their duties, investigate alleged breaches of human rights, and prosecute perpetrators.

European Convention on Human Rights

Alongside the developing UN human rights system, regional assemblies were formed to pursue human rights more effectively. Of these the European has been by far the most effective. It was formed in 1949 by 10 western European countries as the Council of Europe. Six of them separately set up the economic and political organisation that became the European Union (EU). Other western states (and Turkey) joined, and the system proved its worth when Greece was suspended from the organisation in 1969 following a military coup. Over the last 10 years, most of the countries of the former communist bloc have joined the Council of Europe, which has increased the challenges.

The European Convention on Human Rights (ECHR) was signed in 1950 and came into force in 1953. Its main text focuses on civil and political rights (see Box 3.1). The European Court of Human Rights was instituted to enforce it (this is not the same as the European Court of Justice, which is an EU organ). The Court has one judge appointed by each Member State. The ECHR has been a dynamic instrument and there have been 13 protocols since its inception. Some of them have added new rights, the others changing the administration of the system. Additionally, the way the rights themselves are interpreted has changed over the years.

The Human Rights Act (HRA) was enacted in 1998 to incorporate the provisions of the ECHR into British domestic legislation. Until then, the only course available to a British resident who felt that his or her rights had been infringed was to go to the Court in Strasbourg, a slow and expensive process. Since October 2000, the UK courts have been able to apply the provisions of the ECHR. The equivalent provisions for Scotland and Northern Ireland were included in the relevant devolution legislation. The HRA did not create any new rights, but it made the pre-existing rights more readily enforceable. The European Court of Human Rights remains the final arbiter of disputes about the application of the ECHR.

Box 3.1 Human Rights Act, 1998.

The HRA incorporates
- Articles 2–12 and 14 of the ECHR
- Articles 1–3 of the First Protocol
- Articles 1 and 2 of the Sixth Protocol
- Articles 16–18 of the Convention

ECHR
Article 2: right to life
Article 3: prohibition of torture
Article 4: prohibition of slavery and forced labour
Article 5: right to liberty
Article 6: right to a fair trial
Article 7: no punishment without law
Article 8: respect for private and family life
Article 9: freedom of thought, conscience and religion
Article 10: freedom of expression
Article 11: freedom of assembly and association
Article 12: right to marry
Article 14: prohibition of discrimination

First protocol
Article 1: right to protection of property
Article 2: right to education
Article 3: right to free elections

Sixth protocol
Article 1: abolition of death penalty
Article 2: exception to the abolition of death penalty in time of war

Convention
Article 16: restriction on political activity of aliens
Article 17: prohibition of abuse of rights
Article 18: limitation on use of restrictions of rights

Cultural relativism

Some non-western commentators have sought to reject the application of human rights standards on the basis that what they represent are western concepts, and are incompatible with the value systems of other cultures. However, the UDHR was drafted by experts from many countries, covering all regions of the world. Subsequent meetings have agreed the universality and indivisibility of human rights. That is not to say that there is no room for interpretation and application of human rights instruments. The rights are drafted very broadly, and different cultures are bound to apply them differently. However, most people in the world, irrespective of nationality, aspire to live in a state in which they cannot be arbitrarily killed, tortured or held in slavery.

Right to health

The specifics of the right to health have been increasingly debated in recent years. The right itself is enshrined in Article 25 of the UDHR, and expanded in Article 12 of the ICESCR:

1. The States Parties to the present Covenant recognise the right of every-one to the enjoyment of the highest attainable standard of physical and mental health.
2. The steps to be taken by the States Parties to the present Covenant to achieve the full realisation of this right shall include those necessary for:
   (a) The provision for the reduction of the still-birth rate and of infant mortality and for the healthy development of the child;
   (b) The improvement of all aspects of environmental and industrial hygiene;
   (c) The prevention, treatment and control of epidemic, endemic, occupational and other diseases;
   (d) The creation of conditions which would assure to all medical serv-ice and medical attention in the event of sickness.

In the late 1940s, when the UDHR was written, medical care as we know it was in its infancy. Antibiotics were only just starting to be used on a widespread basis, and few clinical investigations were possible. In that context, a right to treatment services would have been meaningless. Even in the early 1960s, there were few treatments for heart attacks or cancer. Thus 'medical attention in the event of sickness' was almost an afterthought. The focus, rightly, was on prevention of infectious diseases, of diseases caused by work, and of those caused by environmental conditions such as overcrowding.

The Article requires the 'highest attainable standard' of health. This is a realistic approach, knowing that resource-poor states cannot achieve the same standards as wealthier ones in the short term. What it does require is that states should do everything they can to create the conditions in which sickness can be prevented (or at least not make them worse), and to provide facilities for all. Article 2 of the ICESCR requires that states should work towards 'achieving progressively' the rights in the Covenant, and that they should co-operate to this end.

It also requires that the rights will be exercised without discrimination of any kind.

However, the right to health is one of the economic, social and cultural groups. Its supervision is left to the UN Commission on Human Rights, which hears reports by states every five years. It can be very critical, for example of states that divert money from healthcare into defence, or that provide services for urban elites at the expense of the rural population, but few people get to hear about this.[9]

In 2002, for the first time, a Special Rapporteur, Professor Paul Hunt, was appointed by the Commission to focus on the right to health. Like the other Special Rapporteurs in the UN system, this post is poorly resourced, and it remains to be seen how much of an impact this will be able to have on the issue.

International humanitarian law

Following his experiences helping the wounded after the Battle of Solferino in 1859, Henri Dunant set up the organisation that became the International Committee of the Red Cross (ICRC). Amongst many other activities, they facilitated conferences between states that agreed the standards with which the military must comply during armed conflict. Those currently in effect are the four Geneva Conventions of 1949, which include the amelioration of the condition of the sick and wounded in the battlefield and at sea, the treatment of prisoners of war, and the protection of the civilian population in time of war. The First Additional Protocol covers a wide range of issues including the prohibition of the use of weapons that will cause 'superfluous injury or unnecessary suffering', or that will cause widespread, long-term and severe damage to the natural environment.[10] Common Article 3 of the four 1949 Conventions gave protection to times of undeclared war, internal armed conflicts, and civil strife, and this was extended by the Second Additional Protocol of 1977.

For the healthcare professional, this gives considerable protection to those engaged, as non-combatants, in the treatment of the victims of war. Military commanders are charged to protect the public health of the communities in which wars are being fought by not targeting food supplies, water facilities and the shelter of the civilian population without very good reason and by protecting medical facilities and personnel. Those wearing a recognised symbol, such as the red cross or red crescent, must be protected by both sides, and they cannot be forced to give preferential medical treatment to the members of one side rather than another.[11]

HEALTHCARE PROFESSIONALS

How a healthcare professional might come across human rights issues will depend to some extent on where he or she is working and whether there is a regional human rights convention. However, the principles remain the same, of dignity, autonomy, and non-discrimination.

These are important concepts for all healthcare professionals. All patients of any age and capacity can be treated with respect. Even those interventions that patients find embarrassing can be done to minimise the threat to the patient's dignity. Autonomy means always taking the patient's wishes into consideration and, normally, following them. Children can have their opinions taken into consideration, even if the final clinical decision differs from exactly what they want. However, nobody can, for example, operate on a conscious, competent adult without that patient's permission.

A patient would normally discuss with family, friends and community leaders and take their advice into consideration, but the final decision is the patients' and not theirs. For example, in the UK, the courts allowed a clinician to treat a patient in her best interests against her expressed views as it is considered that she was acting because of undue influence by a third party.[12]

Non-discrimination means that healthcare delivery should be based on clinical need rather than on other factors such as ethnicity, religion, gender, whether the person lives in a city or a rural area, wherever in the country she lives, or even if the person is a convicted criminal. This is relevant to the individual healthcare worker, who should treat all patients the same, and to health planners who must allocate resources fairly.

Healthcare professionals may think that they could not be involved in documenting human rights violations, but there are many situations in which a doctor or nurse could find themselves dealing with a patient alleging recent or past ill treatment. These include:

- examining individuals on arrival at an institution of detention
- providing medical treatment services in places of detention
- treatment of those in detention taken to hospital emergency facilities
- medical participation in external visits to detention centres
- treatment of those who have recently been released
- investigation of allegations of torture by those no longer detained.[13]

Generally, applying the standards of human rights will reach the same results as applying those of biomedical ethics. The main area of biomedical ethics from which human rights might differ is that of confidentiality. In medical ethics, confidentiality is paramount. The Hippocratic Oath said:

> Whatever I see or hear, professionally or privately, which ought not to be divulged, I will keep secret and tell no one.

In modern medicine this is a fiction. It has long been the case that medical records must be released to a court following a court order, even if the patient has refused consent for their release. For most people such a risk is so small as to be ignored, and most exceptions are obvious, for example treatment records of victims of assault. However, in *Z v Finland* (see Box 3.2), the European Court of Human Rights said:

> At the same time, the Court accepts that the interests of a patient and the community as a whole in protecting the confidentiality of medical data may be outweighed by the interest in investigation and prosecution of crime and in the publicity of court proceedings, ... where such interests are shown to be of even greater importance.[14]

Dual responsibilities

Dual responsibilities occur when a healthcare professional acts directly on behalf of an employer, and so has ethical and legal responsibilities both to the patient and the employer. This would include those working in the military, in prison health services, as forensic physicians (forensic medical examiners, police surgeons) (see also Chapter 3), in occupational health, and for insurance companies. It is also an issue in some types of private healthcare. Many of these roles involve being directly

---

Box 3.2 Z v Finland.

Z was a Finnish woman whose husband was accused of several sexual offences against other women including attempted manslaughter by rape while knowing himself to be HIV positive. At the time of the rapes he had not been demonstrated conclusively to be HIV positive, but it was alleged that he knew that his wife was HIV positive, and therefore he was very likely to be so as well. In the ensuing court case, Z claimed her right not to give evidence against her husband. However, the public prosecutor demanded that her doctors give evidence in the case, and that relevant medical documents be submitted to the court. The European Court of Human Rights found that the request for disclosure of her medical records was in accordance with the law, for a legitimate aim. However, they found that Z's right to privacy had been breached because news articles about the case had been published the following day that allowed her to be identified and as being HIV positive.

employed by the state, so the possibility of acting in a way that makes the state open to accusations of human rights abuses is clear. In extreme cases, the healthcare professional might even be open to prosecution, for example in the International Criminal Court. In other cases of dual responsibility, the duty to the patient has to be balanced against other responsibilities. Advice is available from national medical associations, such as the British Medical Association.[15] Chapter 3 explains these factors from the point of view of the forensic physician.

Psychiatry

Human rights are particularly relevant in psychiatry when patients are detained against their will. That, compulsory detention and treatment is sometimes necessary is not in dispute, but individuals need protection against this happening arbitrarily. The abuses of psychiatry in Soviet Russia, and allegedly till today in China, remind us that the state, through its healthcare professionals, can misuse these powers. The right not to be detained arbitrarily requires that procedures be followed to ensure that there are no alternatives to the use of compulsory powers. In the *Winterwerp* case, the European Court set three conditions to be met in psychiatric cases that:

- the patient should have been shown reliably to be suffering from mental disorder
- the mental illness should be of a kind or degree to justify compulsory confinement
- the detention continues only for so long as the disorder persists to the necessary degree.[16]

In the ECHR, there is also a right to appeal against being detained to an independent tribunal, which must be timely and seen to be impartial.[17] In the UK, this appeal is to the Mental Health Review Tribunal. (see Chapter 8) Treatment should not, of course, be inhuman or degrading. Constraints on privacy, such as sending and receiving correspondence, should be proportional to the patient's health.

CONCLUSION

Human rights are inherent in individuals and place constraints on states as limits on their possible activities. Some are absolute, such as the right not to be tortured, others are qualified or can be modified in times of emergency. The best systems are enforceable through courts such as the European Court of Human Rights, following whose decisions governments are expected to rectify judgements in individual cases, change laws and pay compensation to those whose rights have been abused. However, most rights are enforced by much weaker mechanisms, if at all. That does not mean that they do not exist, as they carry moral force even when no legal pathway is available.

Both human rights and biomedical ethics come from a similar philosophical framework, so tend to arrive at similar solutions to ethical problems. In some fields of medicine, the human rights of patients are an important part of practise. No healthcare professional should be unaware of human rights.

ACKNOWLEDGEMENTS

I would like to thank Dr Stefania Vergnano, Ellie Smith, and Sherman Carroll for their help in writing this chapter.

REFERENCES

1. Robertson AH and Merrills JG. *Human Rights in the World*. Manchester: Manchester University Press, 1996.
2. Anarchical Fallacies; Being an Examination of the Declaration of Rights Issued during the French Revolution, 1823.
3. G.A. Res. 217(A) III U.N. Doc. A/810.
4. Convention on the Prevention and Punishment of the Crime of Genocide, 1948.
5. Convention against Torture and Other Cruel, Inhuman or Degrading Treatment or Punishment, 1984.
6. Convention on the Elimination of All Forms of Discrimination against Women, 1979.
7. Convention on the Rights of the Child, 1989.
8. Robertson G. *Crimes against Humanity: The Struggle for Global Justice*. London: Allen Lane, 1999.
9. Toebes B. *The Right to Health as a Human Right in International Law*. Antwerp: Intersentia, 1999.
10. First Additional Protocol to the Geneva Conventions, 1977, Article 35.
11. International Committee of the Red Cross. *Basic rules of the Geneva Conventions and Their Additional Protocols*. Geneva: ICRC, 1988.
12. *Re T (adult: refusal of treatment)* 1992, 4 All ER 649.
13. Somerville A, Reyes H and Peel M. Doctors and torture. In Peel M and Iacopino V. *The Medical Documentation of Torture*. London: Greenwich Medical Media, 2002.
14. *Z v Finland*, 1997, ECtHR 9/1996/627/811.
15. British Medical Association. *The Medical Profession and Human Rights: Handbook for a Changing Agenda*. London: Zed Books, 2001.
16. *Winterwerp v The Netherlands* 1979, ECtHR Series A, number 33.
17. *DN v Switzerland* 2001, ECtHR 27154/95.

3

Medical ethics and the forensic physician

Michael Wilks

Reference has been made in Chapter 2 to situations where reduced legal and ethical issues may create potential areas of conflict. This chapter highlights one of these situations and explores the implications of such conflicts. The forensic physician (this term is used to describe the police surgeon or forensic medical examiner) fulfils two roles, which feature in almost all examinations, whether of detainees (prisoners), police officers, or victims. These are therapeutic and forensic.

THE THERAPEUTIC ROLE

The therapeutic role involves a traditional doctor–patient relationship, with all the demands of consent and confidentiality inherent in this relationship. The ethical principles involved will be familiar to any doctor working in primary care or hospital medicine. Information obtained should normally be kept confidential, but may be shared with others in the healthcare team, in this case other forensic physicians who may take care of the patient, a custody or forensic nurse, or any doctor to whom the patient is referred. The extent to which this information is shared depends entirely on a judgement as to what constitutes the best interests of the patient in terms of safe detention. Treatment must be given on the basis of fully informed consent. If this is absent, as in the case of incapacity due to alcohol, drugs, or illness, then the doctor proceeds on the basis of the patient's best interests or implied consent.

In this relationship, it is necessary to remember that the custody officer, who carries responsibility for a detainee's welfare, is effectively a member of the healthcare team, and delegates some of this responsibility to others, such as a police officer or civilian acting as a gaoler. While these persons may not have an established duty of confidentiality to the patient, it will on occasions be necessary to share clinical information with them, and to pass on directions regarding medication. This should be done only if the patient's best interests demand it. The sharing of information not relevant to the detainee's detention is unacceptable, in the same way that it is unacceptable that many criminal records contain information (of dubious accuracy) concerning a patient's drug use or human immunodeficiency virus (HIV) status.

The therapeutic relationship is therefore, in most cases, well defined in terms of its ethical boundaries; those who need to know, and the amount they need to know, can usually be identified without difficulty.

While the foregoing states the ethical position relevant to most therapeutic relationships, it is important to emphasize that no doctor–patient relationship has the benefit of absolute privilege. Disclosure may be required in the public interest, where there is otherwise a risk of serious harm to others, and under the direction of a court.

In some police forces, the doctor may also act in an occupational health role. The ethical basis for this aspect of a forensic physician's work is identical to that of a position within a commercial organization.

Conditions in police stations may be far from satisfactory for the treatment and supervision of such conditions as diabetes, drug withdrawal, and severe alcohol intoxication. Special groups of detainees such as asylum seekers or immigration over-stayers will present difficult challenges. The doctor must always be aware of the need for safety, and ensure that prisoners for whom detention represents an unacceptable risk are removed elsewhere, usually to hospital. This may cause disruption to police procedures, and produce organizational problems, but it is essential that the doctor's judgement in these cases is respected and followed.

THE FORENSIC ROLE

The ethical duties and responsibilities of the doctor acting as a forensic physician are, it has to be said, far from clear, and are in some cases in conflict with established advices and statutes. Issues of consent, confidentiality, record sharing, and privacy are all compromised by the fact that the forensic physician is one example of a doctor having a dual responsibility – other examples include doctors working in the armed forces, in prisons, and in occupational health. A doctor with dual responsibility has a duty of care to a patient that overlaps or conflicts with another duty. In the case of the forensic physician the other responsibility is to the process of justice, and leads to complex relationships with investigating officers, criminal justice departments, the legal professions, and the courts. While normal ethical principles of consent, confidentiality, communication, and disclosure are all relevant to forensic medical practice, they are all modified by the duty to serve the interest of justice.

The independence of the forensic physician, in contractual terms, is essential. The ethical independence, the ability to be both part of, and separate from, the process of investigation of crime, follows from the fact that the doctor (while normally remunerated by a police force) must not have a compromised relationship in terms of clinical freedom, privacy of records, and the ability to act in the interest of both prosecution and defence where circumstances require it. It is essential, therefore, that any doctor working with the police or other body fulfilling a similar role should have a contract that emphasizes this independence. Any healthcare professional in a relationship with an authority in which fundamental ethical principles are undermined by poor consent procedures, inadequate arrangements for privacy and confidentiality, or the sharing of sensitive clinical information in records, is not working in an environment conducive to good ethical practice. Doctors contemplating such a relationship need to be aware of the precise contractual obligations in these important ethical and legal areas.

This independence also brings with it particular responsibilities. In fulfilling the role of independent forensic physician, the doctor must remember that the General Medical Council (GMC), which regulates medical practice in the UK, makes it clear that it is unacceptable for a doctor to allow views about the lifestyle to impair his care to the patient. Many of the patients seen in police custody will have criminal records. It may be apparent to the doctor (but not proven) that the reason for a prisoner's detention is entirely justified. The prisoner may have a chronic drug or alcohol problem. These are irrelevant to the good care of the patient. In fact, if they intrude on the decision-making process, or influence the care given by considerations of 'worth', the entire process is compromised, and justice undermined.

A further point is that the doctor attending a detainee in a police station will normally be the only doctor the patient sees. The Police and Criminal Evidence Act 1984 (PACE) allows any detainee to call a doctor of their own choice, but this option is rarely exercised for reasons of availability and cost, so the doctor attending the detainee must provide a level of clinical and ethical care at least equal to that available within the National Health Services (NHS). Arguably, it should be at a higher level, to reflect the vulnerability and lack of choice of the detainee.

The Human Rights Act 1998 (HRA), incorporated into UK Law in October 2000, sets out in more specific details, the rights of patients, and therefore the duties owed by doctors, in some detail. These do not, however, extend these rights and duties beyond those already relevant, but a general knowledge of the relevant articles of the HRA is desirable. In terms of forensic care they are Article 8, which establishes a right to relevant information, and therefore consent to treatment and Article 14, which requires authorities to act in non-discriminatory ways. Again, the mere fact of detention increases vulnerability to discrimination. While it may be argued that consent in this situation can never be 'fully informed', it is the duty of the doctor to ensure that consent to procedures is not given simply as a means to achieve a benefit, such as release from custody.

The specific issues that impinge on the ethics of the forensic medical examination can be summarized under the headings of consent, confidentiality and privacy, and record keeping.

Consent

The 'gold standard' for consent is that of a fully informed process in which the patient is provided with all relevant information, and is acting free from pressure. While it is debatable whether 'all relevant information' can ever be given to the individual patient, it is certainly true that, by virtue of being detained, the detained patient cannot be acting free from pressure. Whether this pressure materially undermines the ability to give valid consent will be for the doctor to decide, but the forensic physician must always consider whether consent for examination, for the taking of samples, and, in the extreme case, for an intimate search, are invalidated by this pressure. The first requirement, therefore, is for time to explain to the patient the precise role of the forensic physician. Suspicion, resentment, and the tendency to label the doctor as the 'police doctor' are all barriers to this process. The old term of 'police surgeon' has not helped the perception of the forensic physician as an independent agent. The simplest way to introduce oneself to a detainee is as a *doctor*, with its immediate implications for healthcare provision and confidentiality. This type of introduction often allows the consultation to proceed with a more detailed explanation of the doctor's role being easier to provide through regained trust. Then there should follow a simple explanation of the reason for the doctor's presence, couched in language and terminology recognizable by the detainee. This might include the statement, 'I am an independent doctor called to see you by the police. I am here for two reasons: to look after any medical problems you may have, but also to advise the police if you are fit to be detained in the police station, and, if necessary to be interviewed. If you have any injuries, I may note these and pass on an opinion about them to the police. Normally, anything you tell me about your health is entirely confidential. Do you understand, and are there any questions you want to ask me?'

The question then arises as to the form of consent. Although written consent may be desirable, this is not normally necessary; although the fact that consent was sought, and verbally given, should be recorded in private notes. Where there is a request for samples, such as intimate samples, or those taken from suspects or victims of sexual assault, written consent, in a form that makes it clear what samples are being taken, may be advisable; but in the case of detainees, it should be noted that written consent for samples is a requirement of PACE. The doctor may consider, however, that written consent in a custody record, which fulfils the requirement of PACE, is not the same thing as a signature on a consent form for medical intervention.

In the absence of consent, an examination cannot be undertaken. However, the particular situation in which both the detainee and the doctor find themselves warrants special consideration. A detainee who is intoxicated or impaired can be assumed to be willing to have immediately necessary treatment, and this should be provided. In the course of such treatment, the doctor will obviously observe injuries, and discover a number of possible facts relevant to the reason for arrest. These observations should be entered in private notes (see below). A strict observance of confidentiality principles demands that these cannot be disclosed in the form of a statement in the absence of informed consent, which in these types of cases, is clearly absent. Many forensic physicians feel that the balance of interests allows this type of information to be disclosed without returning to a competent detainee for the purpose of consent. It can be argued that relevant information will in any case be disclosed at the behest of a court at a later date. It must be said that there is no firm procedure here; however, it can also be said that there have been no procedures laid against doctors by the GMC in pursuit of a complaint for the breaking of confidentiality in these types of circumstances.

Confidentiality and privacy

Privacy and the preservation of the safety of the doctor are hard to reconcile, especially in circumstances where a detainee is impaired by alcohol, drugs, or mental illness. It is commonly believed that the presence of a chaperone or police officer compromises the confidentiality of a consultation. Although this may be an inhibiting factor on disclosure of sensitive information to the doctor, it is not in itself a risk to the detainee, as it is highly unlikely that information given to the doctor, and overheard, would be passed on, as that information has not been obtained under caution. It is desirable that a chaperone should be present for any examination undertaken by a doctor on a patient, including a police officer, of the opposite sex. If there are issues of personal safety, a police officer should be present, available to intervene, but ideally out of earshot.

Such a useful compromise may be difficult to achieve in some police stations. Whether this simply increases the temperature and makes it more likely that a prisoner will feel threatened, is debatable – as some assaults on doctors have taken place in presence of officers. If an assault does take place, it is likely to be as a result of a lack of caution in not assessing the risk. When in doubt, a prisoner should be observed regarding an assessment of fitness for detention, and a fuller assessment made later when and if the situation allows.

Records

Records made by the forensic physician fall into a number of categories, with varying levels of confidentiality and, therefore, different issues with regard to disclosure. It is important to remember that any record made that then forms part of the custody record will be subject to disclosure under the Criminal Procedures and Investigations Act. Therefore, it is vital for forensic physicians to consider very carefully what it is appropriate to record in the documents that will be shared between various authorities. Many records, such as the *Book 83* used in the Metropolitan Police, have a very limited function. In the case of the examination of a detainee, the doctor needs to record information that is relevant to the safe detention of a patient. This will, therefore, include the need for observations at set time intervals, the provision of medication, fitness for interview, and the need for any medical review. This information is essential to allow the custody officer to fulfil his obligations under PACE. Clinical information that is not relevant to this process should not normally be included in this type of record. In the case of victims of assault, who may include police officers, information relevant to the investigation of a crime should be recorded. This will include a record of injuries, an assessment of an officer's fitness for duty, and, in some cases, an observation as to the consistency of the injuries with the history given (always bearing in mind that at this stage the doctor will have incomplete information about an allegation of assault).

In addition to a formal entry, which may be in a custody record, *Book 83*, or other form, the doctor must keep private records. Though these are called 'private', they do not imply that they are free from an obligation to disclose. These records should be as full as possible, allowing the physician to make an accurate legal statement (often a considerable time after the examination). They should be made contemporaneously, or as soon as possible following the examination. They should not be routinely passed to any third party, and can only be disclosed on the basis of fully informed consent.

Private notes may include sketches, drawings, photographs, and, occasionally video. Whatever form the records are held in, they collectively form a complete private record, subject to the normal rules of disclosure.

FURTHER READING

Confidentiality: Protecting and Providing Information. London: GMC, 2000.

Guidelines for Doctors Asked to Perform Intimate Body Searches. London: BMA, Association of forensic physician (formerly Association of police surgeons) 1999.

Medical Ethics Today. The BMA's Handbook of Ethics and Law, 2nd edition. London: BMJ Books.

Revised Interim Guidelines on Confidentiality for Police Surgeons in England, Wales and Northern Ireland. London: BMA, Association of forensic physician (formerly Association of police surgeons) 1998.

Police and Criminal Evidence Act 1984 Home Office; *Police and Criminal Evidence Act 1984 (Section 60(1)(a) and Section 66(1)) Codes of Practice A–E, Revised Edition.* London: The Stationery Office, 2003; *Police and Criminal Evidence (Northern Ireland) Order 1989,* Northern Ireland Office *Police and Criminal Evidence (Northern Ireland) Order 1989 (Articles 60 and 65) Codes of Practice.* Belfast: HMSO, 1996.

Report of the Home Office Working Group on Police Surgeons, Annex D. London: Home Office, 2001.

Stark M and Norfolk G. *Metropolitan Police Service Good Practice Guidelines for FMEs.* 2002.

The Health Care of Detainees in Police Stations. London: British Medical Association and Association of Forensic Physicians, 2004.

The Impact of the Human Rights Act 1998 on Medical Decision Making. London: BMA, 2000.

4
Confidentiality*

Peter Schütte

Ever since the Hippocratic Oath was first taken 2500 years ago, confidentiality has been recognised by the medical profession as a cornerstone of good clinical practice. In 1947, the Declaration of Geneva (amended in 1968) strongly reinforced the declaration of confidentiality in the Hippocratic Oath. The Declaration states:

> I will respect the secrets which are confided in me, even after the patient has died.

In recent times legal, social, and technological advances have brought increasingly complex obligations and challenges for healthcare professionals who wish to safeguard patient confidentiality. Under the common law, confidentiality may be enforced by a patient through an injunction or with an action for damages in a civil court, but in the absence of any demonstrable harm, it is likely that the damages awarded would be limited, and civil claims are very rare.

A breach of the Data Protection Act 1998 (vide infra) can result in civil or criminal proceedings.

Disciplinary proceedings based on employment law may follow a breach of confidentiality caused by staff working for the National Health Service (NHS) the primary health provider in the UK. If an NHS healthcare worker breaches confidentiality, alternatively or in addition, he or she may be asked to explain and apologise to a complainant under the patients' complaints procedures. This may be as part of local resolution (stage 1), independent review (stage 2) or a Health Service Commissioner's (Ombudsman's) investigation (stage 3).

Caldicott Guardians may scrutinise arrangements for protecting patient confidentiality, as could a hospital inquiry into an adverse incident, a review of clinical performance by an outside body such as a medical royal college, or a performance review by the General Medical Council (GMC). Arrangements for protecting patient confidentiality

may also be appraised under local audit and clinical governance procedures, or nationally by the Commission for Health Improvement.[1]

In practical terms, it most frequently falls to registration bodies
such as the GMC, the General Dental Council (GDC), the Nursing &
Midwifery Council (NMC) and the various boards of the Council for
Professions Supplementary to Medicine to enforce patient confidentiality as an ethical rather than legal matter. No one should underestimate
the vigour with which the registration bodies will pursue an allegation
of breach of confidentiality. Medical practitioners found guilty of serious professional conduct because of a breach of patients' confidentiality may have their names erased from the register, depriving them of
their livelihood.

The registration bodies publish guidelines on confidentiality and all
registered practitioners should study these carefully and review them
when they are updated.[2,3,4]

DISCLOSURE TO THE PATIENT

It is common practice for practitioners to agree to the disclosure of a
patient's full records to the patient (or the patient's legal representative)
on demand. However, in 1994 the Court of Appeal held that patients do
not have an unconditional right of access to their clinical records at common law. A former psychiatric patient requested access to his records,
but on medical advice full disclosure was refused on the grounds that it
would be detrimental to his health.[5] The GMC says that when a doctor is
satisfied that it is appropriate for the information to be released, the doctor should provide the information promptly.

The Data Protection Act 1998 regulates the processing of information
about individuals including the obtaining, use or disclosure of information. It recognises individuals' rights to be told what information is being
processed about them and to have it disclosed under certain restrictions.
The Act covers paper and computer records without time limit.

The basic data protection principles of the Act give data subjects and
data users certain responsibilities and rights. These includes the following.

Responsibilities

Personal data shall

- be obtained and processed fairly and lawfully
- be held only for specified purposes
- not be used or disclosed in any other way or for any other purpose

- be adequate, relevant and not excessive in relation to the purpose for which they are held
- be accurate and kept up to date
- not be kept longer than is necessary
- be processed according to the rights of data subjects
- be held secure.

Rights

Data subjects are entitled to

- be told that data is held about them and of the purposes for which their data will be processed
- have access to the data
- have the data corrected when inaccurate.

Under the Data Protection (Subject Access Modification) (Health) Order 2000 (SI 2000 no 413), information may be exempt from the subject access provisions of the Data Protection Act 1998 on the grounds that disclosure would be likely to cause serious harm to the physical or mental health or condition of the data subject or any other person. The regulations stipulate that it is the healthcare professional involved in the patient's care who should be consulted to advise whether this exemption applies.

Disclosure can also be resisted if it may cause a breach of confidentiality to a third party who is not a healthcare professional.[6]

The Access to Medical Reports Act 1988 covers information contained in reports produced by a doctor providing care for a patient. It does not cover situations where there is no established doctor–patient relationship (for example reports by occupational health physicians who do not provide clinical care).

The Access to Health Records Act 1990 applies only after the death of the patient.

The NHS Venereal Diseases Regulations 1974 enforce the confidentiality of all information given by and about patients with venereal diseases who attend genito-urinary clinics. Information that may identify the patient may not be disclosed except to treat or prevent the disease. This means that a patient's GP may not be told unless the patient agrees to this disclosure. Case notes from these clinics are kept separately from other hospital records. Similar restrictions on disclosure of information in relation to patients examined or treated for any sexually transmitted disease are contained in the NHS and Primary Care Trusts (Sexually Transmitted Diseases) Directions 2000.

The Human Fertilisation and Embryology Act 1990 gives a high degree of protection against disclosure of information. Any disclosure outside the exemptions may be a criminal offence, punishable by a maximum of two years imprisonment and a fine.

When a practitioner is the subject of a complaint or litigation, disclosure to the patient is usually carried out with the assistance of the practitioner's medical defence organisation (MDO). The consent of other practitioners who have written in the notes is not necessary.

DISCLOSURE TO THIRD PARTIES

When a patient gives consent to disclosure to a third party (preferably in writing), the practitioner may agree to do so in strict accordance with that consent. For consent to be valid, the patient must understand

- to whom the information will be disclosed
- what will be disclosed
- the purpose of the disclosure
- significant, foreseeable consequences of the disclosure
- that in certain circumstances, such as disclosure to an insurance company or employers, relevant information cannot be concealed or withheld.

If the practitioner has any doubt about the validity of the consent, he should confirm that the patient understands the points raised above and their implications.

Disclosure to a third party contrary to the patient's wishes should only take place in the most exceptional circumstances, for example where the health, safety or welfare of someone may otherwise be placed at serious risk.

DISCLOSURE WITHOUT THE CONSENT OF THE PATIENT

Disclosure to relatives and others caring for the patient

Information is often shared with a patient's relatives or other persons helping to care for the patient. This may be without the patient's authority, but only where it is clearly in the patient's best medical interests to do so. This situation most frequently occurs with terminally ill patients.

Normally a practitioner will disclose all relevant information concerning a young child to parents. Where parents are divorced, information may still be disclosed to either parent unless a court has removed parental responsibility from one parent. It is important that where information is given to a parent or a parent's solicitors, the confidentiality of the other parent is not compromised and this may be achieved by removing any information about the other parent before passing on a copy of the notes.

Children over 16 should enjoy the same rights to confidentiality as adults. This right may be inferred from the provisions of the Family Law Reform Act 1969 which enables children of 16 and over to consent to medical treatment.

For children under 16, consent to disclosure will depend on whether or not the child is 'Gillick competent' (see below). Following a Department of Health (DoH) publication which set out certain circumstances in which contraceptive devices could be provided to persons under the age of 16 without parental consent, Mrs Victoria Gillick, herself the mother of young children sought a court ruling in 1983 that the guidance in the publication was unlawful. The case went as far as the House of Lords, which ruled in favour of the DoH.[7] The ruling gave rise to the concept of so-called 'Gillick competence' where a child's maturity and understanding is sufficient to enable an appreciation of what is involved. The practitioner should ordinarily respect the wishes of a 'Gillick competent' child to confidentiality, after making every reasonable effort to persuade the child to involve the parents or guardians. There will be rare occasions when, in the practitioner's judgement, it is in the 'Gillick competent' child's best interests to disclose information against the child's wishes. If the practitioner decides to disclose information to a parent, legal guardian or social services through the child protection team for example, contrary to the child's wishes, then he should, with very rare exceptions, inform the child in advance of his intentions. If a child under 16 is not 'Gillick competent', then a parent or legal guardian ought to be kept fully informed about any consultation, but it is possible, extremely rare occasions on that it is not in the child's best interests to do so, in which case social services or an equivalent authority may have to be informed instead.

Disclosure to other healthcare professionals

Clinical information is normally shared by a practitioner with other healthcare professionals involved in the care of a particular patient without the patient's express consent and on a 'need to know' basis. Patients should be made aware that personal information will be shared within the healthcare team, and any objection must be respected, except where this would put others at risk of serious harm or death. The doctor has a duty to be satisfied that all members of staff are aware of their obligation to preserve confidentiality.

A practitioner who is the subject of complaint is not entitled to have access to clinical notes, made by a colleague relating to the care of the patient after the events giving rise to the complaint, without the consent of the patient.

Disclosure as a statutory requirement

Under the Public Health (Control of Disease) Act 1984 and various regulations a doctor must notify certain infectious diseases.

A doctor or midwife present at a birth must notify the relevant authority within 36 hours. A doctor treating a patient who dies must give the cause of death on the death certificate (NHS Notification of Births and Deaths Regulations 1974). It is unlawful to omit conditions from the certificate that the doctor knows, contributed to death, such as Human Immunodeficiency Virus (HIV) infection, however distressing this may be for the relatives of the deceased.

Under the Abortion Act 1967, and the Abortion Regulations 1991, a doctor terminating a pregnancy must notify this to the Chief Medical Officer of the Department of Health.

The Health Service (Control of Patient Information) Regulations 2002 were made under the provisions of the Health and Social Care Act 2001. They enable the flow of clinical information, with or without patient consent, within and from the NHS with regard to:

1 Cancer registries
2 Communicable diseases and other risks to public health and
3 Medical purposes such as medical audit and research.

At present this is an enabling legislation and there is no compulsion on a practitioner to disclose information under the provisions of the Health and Social Care Act 2001.

Disclosure to employers and insurance companies

The Access to Medical Reports Act 1988 provides that, when a patient requires it, employers and insurance companies may not be shown a report by a doctor who has seen the patient for clinical purposes, until the patient has seen the report and given consent for its disclosure.

Occupational physicians have dual loyalties, both to their patients and to their employers. Where a firm provides a clinical service as a 'perk' for employees, it should be understood by the employer that the practitioner owes the patient the usual obligation of confidentiality.

Disclosure to social services and the police

Where a registered practitioner has reason to suspect child abuse he will have an ethical obligation to volunteer information to an appropriate authority, such as Social Services. Only in very rare circumstances, where a doctor feels it is in the patient's best medical interests, will the doctor withhold information.

Information which is given should be provided on a strictly 'need-to-know' basis. Ultimately, the onus is on the practitioner, and not the recipient of the information, to decide what is, and what is not needed.

The Road Traffic Act 1988 places a duty upon any person to tell the police on request the name and address of a person who is alleged to be guilty of offences under the Act. However, such disclosure should not include clinical information.

Normally, the fact that a patient is a patient is itself strictly confidential information. However, if a patient commits an offence such as an assault against a healthcare professional or his staff, this need not prevent a healthcare professional from seeking the protection of the police where appropriate. Disclosure to the police should be kept to a minimum and be limited to information necessary for the protection of the practitioner or his colleagues. It is unlikely to include any significant clinical information.

There is no legal obligation on any citizen to volunteer information to the police concerning a crime. An exception to this involves terrorism, which includes the threat or use of violence for political ends and any use of violence for the purposes of putting the public or any section of the public in fear.

There are circumstances, albeit rare, where a breach of confidentiality may be justified on the grounds that failure to do so may place the patient or some other person at risk of serious harm or death.

In the case of Tarasoff v Regents of University of California[8] a psychiatrist was successfully sued after he had failed to warn the girlfriend of one of his patients that he knew her life was in danger. The patient later murdered the girl. No similar case has occurred in the UK and it is a matter of debate whether the UK courts would take the same view.

However, in the English case of W v Egdell (1989)[9] a claim was brought for damages against a consultant psychiatrist. He had examined a violent patient who was hoping to be released from detention under the Mental Health Act 1983, at the request of the patient's solicitors. The psychiatrist was so concerned by his findings that he disclosed a copy of his report to the appropriate authorities without the consent of the patient. As a consequence, the patient's application for release was turned down.

A judge dismissed the claim and his decision was upheld by the Court of Appeal on the grounds that the doctor had acted in the public interest.

A healthcare professional may not necessarily be able to justify the voluntary disclosure of medical information to the police in relation to serious crime, if the crime is non-violent or if the suspect is already in custody and can be prosecuted successfully with the information already available. Refusal by a healthcare professional to answer questions need not obstruct the police in their enquiries.

Forensic physicians (forensic medical examiners, police surgeons) may find themselves in a particularly difficult situation arising from their dual role as personal clinicians to detainees in a police cell on the one hand, and gatherers of forensic evidence for the police on the other hand.[3] (see Chapter 3) Their duty of medical confidentiality to a detainee is no different from that of any other doctor to his patient.

Forensic physicians are not obliged to disclose detainee's treatment records routinely to the custody officer without the detainee's consent. These records are not regarded as 'unused material', as defined in the Criminal Procedure and Investigations Act 1996, because under this Act, the forensic physician is not part of the investigation team.

Forensic physicians should consider carefully any proposed contractual obligation placed on them by an employing police authority to disclose their clinical records as a matter of routine to police personnel without prior and informed consent of the detainee. This can be important because some detainees may be drunk, under the influence of drugs, or suffering from psychosis for example, and temporarily lack capacity to give or withhold consent to the disclosure of clinical information to the police at the time they are seen.

Under the Police Reform Act 2002, consent to process a blood sample taken when the patient lacked capacity must be obtained after the detainee recovers capacity to consent in order for the sample to be analysed. The same principles apply to disclosure of clinical information.[10]

However, the forensic physician does have a contractual obligation to tell the police if the detainee is fit to be detained, fit to be interviewed and fit for trial, and also to provide such medical information as will enable the police to properly care for the detainee, in the detainee's best medical interest.

Disclosure to the courts

A healthcare professional who is asked to breach confidentiality in court must ask the judge or presiding officer for permission to breach confidentiality, but if directed to answer a question, may be found in contempt of court if he fails to do so. A healthcare professional may be summoned to court and compelled to produce confidential documents subject to the judge's directions.

Disclosure to the coroner

A healthcare professional normally requires the authority of a deceased patient's executors, or where the patient died intestate, the next of kin, before disclosing information. However, the coroner has powers to investigate the circumstance of a death, and clinical notes and relevant information must be disclosed to the coroner or coroner's officer on request to enable the coroner to determine whether an inquest should be held and the conduct of the inquest.

Disclosure for medical teaching, research, audit, and administration

Medical information for use in teaching, research, and audit is normally kept anonymous to preserve confidentiality. Where it may be possible to identify an individual, the patient concerned should be made aware of the possibility and given the opportunity to withhold consent to disclosure. Exceptions apply, as above, under the provisions of the Health & Social Care Act 2001.

Where medical information identifiable to an individual is disclosed for administrative purposes, the healthcare professional should be satisfied that administrative staff are aware of their own duty of confidentiality, whether such staff work within the NHS or not.

CONCLUSION

The different priorities of medicine and the law make it difficult to resolve all of the dilemmas which can arise from medical confidentiality. Healthcare professionals in doubt whether or not to disclose information without a patient's consent should not hesitate to contact a medical defence organisation or professional association for expert advice. The future is unlikely to see a simplification of the ethical or legal issues.

REFERENCES

1. Department of Health. *Guidance to the Commission for Health Improvement on Obtaining and Disclosing Information under the Health Act*, London, 1999.

2. General Medical Council. *Confidentiality: Protecting and Providing Information.* London, 2000.
3. General Dental Council. *Maintaining Standards: Guidance to the Dental Team on Professional and Personal Conduct,* London, 2000.
4. Nursing & Midwifery Council. *Code of Professional Conduct.* London, 2002.
5. *R v Mid Glamorgan* Family Health Service Authority and Others, ex parte Martin, 1995, 1 All ER 356.
6. The Information Commissioner. *Use and Disclosure of Health Data,* London, 2002.
7. *Gillick v West Norfolk and Wisbech* Health Authority, 1985. 3 All ER 402.
8. *Tarasoff v Regents of the University of California,* 529 P 2d 5S (Cal, 1974); 551 P 2d 334 (Cal, 1976).
9. *W v Edgell,* 1989, 1 All ER 835, 849.

FURTHER READING

Hoyte PJ. *Can I see the records?* London: MDU Services Ltd, 2000.
McLean S, Mason, SR. Legal and Ethical Aspects of Heathcare. Greenwich Medical Media, London 2003.
Mason JK, McCall Smith A. *Law and medical ethics,* 5th edn. London: Butterworths, 1999.
Schütte P. *Confidentiality,* London: MDU Services Ltd, 2001.

5

Consent to medical treatment

Ian Wall

Non-consensual physical contact forms the basis of the criminal offence of assault and the civil wrong of battery; laws which affirm principles that seek to ensure preservation of individual integrity and the inviolability of the body.[1]

In addition to legitimising otherwise illegal acts of contact, consent, as a reflection of choice, lies behind ethical notions of individual autonomy and self-determination.

A respect for these principles should form the basis of good medical practise, rather than outdated ideas of medical paternalism exemplified by the maxim 'doctor knows best', which often resulted in the relegation of therapeutic consent to paper exercises.

VALID CONSENT

Whether an individual is able to give consent, and whether indeed such consent is 'true' or legally valid is dependant on three factors. The individual must have sufficient *capacity*, they must possess sufficient understanding or *knowledge* of the proposed intervention, and their agreement to undergo the proposed treatment must be *voluntary*, that is, it must be freely given and not tainted by any degree of coercion or undue influence, either from the healthcare professional or family members.[2]

CAPACITY

There is a legal presumption that any person over the age of 18 who is not suffering from a mental incapacity (infra) is capable of giving consent for, or refusing, medical treatment,[2] unless there is evidence to the contrary.[3]

An individual will only be regarded as having sufficient capacity to consent if able to comprehend and retain information material to the particular treatment, as well as the consequences of non-treatment. Furthermore, the individual must believe the information provided, and must be in a position to assess, or weigh up this information to arrive at a decision.[4]

The concept of capacity emphasises the decision-making *process* within the context of the particular decision the individual purports to make, and not the decision itself. Thus capacity must be commensurate with the gravity of the decision; the more complex the decision, so the greater the capacity required to make it.[5]

The assessment of an individual's capacity to engage in therapeutic decision-making falls, in the first instance, to the treating clinician, assisted by professional guidance[6] relating to the clinical and social factors that require consideration. Ultimately, however, a decision on the capacity of any particular individual is a question of law and a matter to be decided by the courts.

An adult's decision-making ability may be impaired by a variety of mental and/or physical factors; enduring factors such as severe intellectual impairment, temporary factors such as childhood or acute mental illness, or the transient effects of unconsciousness, fear, or intoxication.

Whatever the level of capacity, however, individuals should, as far as practicable, be given the opportunity to participate in any therapeutic decision-making process.

Adults

Adults lacking capacity

There are currently no provisions in England and Wales under which another individual, be it family, next of kin, or the courts may give or withhold consent on behalf of an adult who lacks capacity.[7]

Administering medical treatment in the absence of consent would ordinarily constitute an unlawful act, exposing the treating practitioner to legal censure but also potentially depriving incapable individuals of the medical care they require. In these circumstances treatment may be justified under the common law principle of necessity, and any such treatment may be lawful, provided it is in the patient's 'best interests'.

In Re F[8] the court, faced with an application to sterilise a seriously mentally disabled adult female, stated that, in general, treatment would be in the person's best interests;

> if, but only if it is carried out in order either to save life or to ensure improvement or prevent deterioration in their physical or mental health.

The concept of best interests is, in this respect, capable of being broadly defined, and could be utilised to justify most types of therapeutic intervention.

In addition, the court adopted the peer-group test laid down in Bolam[9] as the appropriate standard for assessing 'best interests', as well as what was 'necessary'. This approach has attracted considerable criticism because these principles, when viewed in combination, appear to concentrate decision-making power in the hands of the medical profession allowing them, rather than the judges, to define the limits of the legal defence of necessity.

More recently, however, the courts have extended the concept of best interests into social, cultural, and religious dimensions, so that it no longer equates to best *medical* interests.[10] The Bolam test still remains relevant, however, in allowing the court to assess the acceptability of treatment options advocated in individual cases.

The dictates of good medical practise now reflect this judicial holism, and while routine treatment decisions remain the province of the clinical team in charge of the patients care, an exploration of individual patient's pre-morbid beliefs, values and feelings form an essential ingredient of the assessment process.

Where the proposed treatment is contentious, such as non-therapeutic sterilisation, or withdrawal of artificial treatment, or where there is a dispute over issues of best interests, any decision will require the sanction of the court.

In Scotland, statutory provisions allow for the appointment of proxies to look after the welfare of incapacitated individuals over the age of 16, and to consent to medical treatment on their behalf where appropriate.[11]

Emergency treatment in adults

In Re F[12] the court recognised the qualitative differences between 'elective' treatment in circumstances where the patient has suffered a permanent loss of capacity and emergency treatment involving a temporary loss of capacity. In the latter situation, the doctrine of necessity is strictly limited to treatment that is 'reasonably required' in the best interests of the patient. Any further or additional interventions should, where possible (or reasonable), be postponed pending recovery of competence, however inconvenient that may be.[13]

Mental illness and the Mental Health Act 1983

Individuals suffering from a psychiatric illness should not automatically be regarded as incapable of consenting to medical treatment. This is equally true in respect of those hospitalised both on a formal and a voluntary basis.

Individuals suffering from a defined mental disorder who are the subject of formal detention may be treated without their consent within the confines of s63 of the Mental Health Act 1983. While the form of 'treatment' permissible has been widely interpreted and extends beyond routine psychiatric treatment,[14] any such treatment must be strictly in respect of the patient's psychiatric condition and not a related physical condition. Additional statutory protection exists in respect of non-consensual treatment relating to electro-convulsive therapy (ECT) and 'psychosurgery'.[15]

Refusal of treatment (adults)

As logic would dictate, the law also recognises the absolute and inviolable right of an individual not to be treated against their will.[16] A competent adult has the right to refuse medical treatment, even where a refusal appears irrational or ultimately life threatening,[3] and refusals that may appear unreasonable to the healthcare professional should not automatically be equated with a lack of capacity.

Where, however, the refusal appears profoundly irrational, or where temporary clinical factors are believed to have reduced the patient's capacity, or where the patient has an insufficiency of information on the consequences of his or her refusal, the practitioner should seek further guidance from the court concerning the validity of the refusal.[17]

The court's continued affirmation of general ethical principles of inviolability and self-determination may appear simple in theory, though a strict practical application of these principles is often more problematic, particularly in the face of third party interests; as illustrated by Re S and Re MB.[2,17] Both cases involve the refusal of pregnant women to consent to Caesarean section. In both cases the courts voiced explicit support for the foregoing principles but in both cases the refusals were overridden on grounds of capacity. The decisions have been criticised for manipulating the fluid concept of capacity rather than addressing influential policy issues affecting others or society at large.[18]

Advance directives, anticipatory declarations, living wills

These are statements made in advance of the occurrence of, and dependant on, the development of a medical condition. They are contingent refusals made by competent individuals in anticipation of possible future incompetence, and they seek to provide direction to healthcare professionals in either a general or specific area (such as refusals of blood transfusion in Jehovah's Witnesses).

In any event, the legitimacy of such directives has found support from the General Medical Council and the professional defence bodies[26] who state that advanced directives should be respected and binding on the healthcare professional if valid. Validity will depend on whether such directives were clearly established, applicable to the case in hand, and free from undue influence.

Withdrawal of medical treatment

The 'best interests' test was approved in respect of withdrawal of treatment in persistent vegetative states (PVS)[20] and in respect of medical conditions that carry a bleak prognosis.[21]

Where a body of medical opinion believes that treatment (such as artificial feeding) is futile, and no longer of benefit to the patient, it can be stopped as its continuation would no longer be in the patient's best interest.

The withdrawal of medical treatment raises issues of sanctity of life, issues which Article 2 of the European Convention on Human Rights[22] seek to protect. Article 2 does not, however, appear to impose an obligation to treat if the burden of such treatment far outweighs the benefits. Furthermore, Article 2 should be viewed in light of Article 3, which seeks to protect an individual from inhumane and degrading treatment, which it has been held includes the right to die with dignity.

The USA has chosen to follow a different approach in dealing with individuals who are artificially maintained, in the form of the principle of 'substituted judgement'.[23] This, essentially, is a legal fiction whereby a proxy (usually a judge) considers the desirability of any treatment by viewing it from the patient's perspective.

Consent to medical treatment in minors[24]

16 to 17 years of age

Under section 8 of the Family Law Reform Act 1969,[25] individuals aged 16 and 17 years (subject to satisfying the general principles in relation to valid consent outlined above) are entitled to consent to medical (and dental) treatment, without reference to those exercising parental responsibility.

In circumstances involving hazardous or complex treatments, good practise dictates the involvement of parents or carers, unless the young person refuses.[26] This consent cannot be overridden by those exercising parental control but can be overridden by the court.

The under 16s

The capacity of children below the age of 16 to consent to medical treatment depends on whether the child has achieved a sufficient understanding and intelligence to appreciate the purpose, nature, consequences, and risks of a particular treatment (as well as failure to treat), and that he (or she) has the ability to appraise the medical advice. This developmental concept which became known as 'Gillick' competence,[27] is dependant on the child's chronological age, mental age, and emotional maturity, and is a recognition of a child's increasing autonomy with advancing age.

The treating practitioner is entrusted with deciding whether a child is competent and whether the treatment proposed is in the child's best interests,[28] and, if of the opinion that the child is competent, the practitioner may proceed without the need to obtain additional 'parental' consent.

In the interests of good practise the practitioner should, however, seek to persuade the child to inform his or her parents in respect of the proposed treatment.

In Scotland, the 'Gillick' ruling has been placed on a statutory footing.[29]

Refusal of treatment (minors)

Competent minors under the age of 18 may refuse treatment, though their wishes may be over-ruled by a person exercising parental responsibility, or the courts. In Re R[30] the court found that a 15-year old ward of court suffering from mental health problems was not competent to refuse medical treatment. The court expressed the view that even if the minor had been 'Gillick' competent the court (or parent) would have had the power to overrule the decision to refuse treatment. The court held that the power to consent and the power to refuse were qualitatively different; the former required the agreement of either party whereas an exercise of the latter power required both parties to refuse.

In Re W,[31] a 16-year old who refused compulsory feeding for anorexia nervosa, was deemed competent though the court held that the Family Law Reform Act (FLRA) did not address the issue of refusals and therefore did not prevent the court from authorising treatment on the child's behalf.

Where treatment is initiated against the child's wishes it is usually restricted to cases where the treatment is in the child's best interests and where the child is at grave risk without treatment.[32] The highly individual nature of these cases usually requires an application to the court for a ruling on the legality of embarking on a course of treatment.

Children and young persons lacking capacity

Treating incompetent children requires the consent of those exercising parental responsibility, and such treatment needs to be in the child's best interests.

Where those exercising parental responsibility refuse to consent on behalf of the child, and that refusal runs contrary to reasonable medical practise as well as the best interests (in the wider sense) of the child, it may be over-ruled by the courts. Similarly a doctor is not required to carry out treatment *under* parental wishes unless the treatment proposed is in the child's best interests.[33]

Parental responsibility

The Children Act 1989 (see Chapter 15) defines the legal concept of parental responsibility as;

> all rights, duties, powers, responsibilities and authority which by law a parent has in relation to the child ...

In practise this includes one or more of the following: the child's parents (if married at the time of birth), the mother (but not the father) in the case of the unmarried, a legally appointed guardian, or the local authority. The rights granted under the Act will decline accordingly as the child matures to adulthood.

In any event, the child should be kept informed and engaged in respect of their treatment or proposed treatment and their views sought as a matter of good practise.

Emergency treatment of children

In circumstances where a competent child refuses treatment and the exigencies of time make it impractical to contact those with parental authority or the courts, the courts have suggested that treatment should be directed in favour of preserving life.

KNOWLEDGE AND THE SUFFICIENCY OF INFORMATION

A failure to provide adequate information or to disclose any attendant risks of a proposed treatment may potentially vitiate consent thereby exposing the practitioner to an allegation of battery. The courts have, however, indicated that battery is an inappropriate remedy in this context,[34] regarding negligence instead as the correct legal action.

The duty to inform, advise, and warn of risks is one aspect of the general duty of care practitioners owe to their patients. For consent to be legally valid, the patient needs only to understand the purpose of the procedure in broad terms.[35]

In Sidaway,[34] the plaintiff had suffered the consequences of a risk inherent in her treatment, a risk of which she had not been informed. She argued that she should have received a full and detailed account of the procedure and should have been warned of all possible risks inherent in the treatment.

The majority of the House of Lords confirmed that the test of liability in respect of a doctor's duty to warn of inherent risks in treatment was that laid down in Bolam,[9] that is the quality and quantity of the information provided to a patient, including risk warnings, was a matter of clinical judgement. There is no liability provided a practitioner can demonstrate that he has acted in accordance with a practise accepted at the time as proper by a responsible body of medical opinion in relation to what information was provided and what was not.

As a matter of law, the court retained the right to overrule medical opinion on disclosure of particular risks where they were obviously necessary for any informed choice.

The majority of the court rejected Mrs Sidaway's contention and concluded that English law did not recognise the doctrine of informed consent (though a minority opinion did, however, provide some support for the principal of full disclosure).

Informed consent has found favour in other common law jurisdictions[36] and in these circumstances therefore, it is the courts that set the standards of disclosure and not the profession. Individual patients must be provided with information on all 'material' or significant risks involved in their treatment.

In this respect the US courts have adopted the 'reasonable patient' or 'prudent patient' test (rather than the 'reasonable doctor' test which is employed in the UK).

"A risk is material when a reasonable person, in what the physician knows or should know to be the patient's position, would be likely to attach significance to the risk or the cluster of risks in deciding whether or not to forgo the proposed therapy"[37]

Under this test, the duty to inform depends on 'materiality', and this is assessed by reference to whether a reasonable person in the patient's position would be likely to attach significance to the risk. The 'character' of the risk, therefore, if considerable importance and so a relatively minor risk that has some special significance for an individual patient (so called 'special' risks)[38] is more likely to be elevated to the status of materiality. In any event, materiality is a matter of law, for the court to decide.

The precedents set by Bolam and Sidaway represent the current law in the UK in relation to the quantity and quality of information provided when eliciting consent. Of late, however, the courts have appeared to adopt a more 'patient-centred' approach,[39,40] alongside a greater willingness to examine the logic of medical opinion.

Furthermore, professional standards and advice on disclosure of risks are currently more stringent than the legal standards set out in Bolam and Sidaway.[41]

FORM OF CONSENT

It is not a legal requirement to acquire written consent for medical or surgical procedures,[42] though it is regarded as a good practise to do so.

Consent may be express or implied. An example of implied consent would be a patient offering his arm for venepuncture, and in practise reliance is placed on this form of consent in most minor interventions. Where the proposed intervention is more complex, however, an express or explicit form of consent requiring the patient to make a positive statement should be obtained.

Such a positive statement may be oral or written. It is in the latter form that consent is evidenced in major interventions but it is the quality of the explanation given and the information imparted which is important and not the signature at the bottom of a standard consent form. A signed consent form should not be regarded as a legal disclaimer.

REFERENCES AND NOTES

1. See generally Michael Davis, *Textbook on Medical Law*, 2nd edn, Chapter 6, Blackstone Press, UK, on the ethical and legal dimensions of consent.
2. *Re MB*, 1997, 38 BMLR 175; 1997 2 FCR 541. Court overriding refusal of a patient to undergo a Caesarian section due to a needle phobia.
3. *Re T (Adult: Refusal of Medical Treatment)*, 1992, 4 All ER 649 CA. 9 BMLR per Lord Donaldson.
4. *Re C (Adult: Refusal of Medical Treatment)*, 1994, 1 All ER 819. Re MB 1997, 38 BMLR 175.
5. *Re T*, 1992, 3 WLR 782 at 799 per Lord Donaldson who suggested in the case of refusals a risk-related standard where competence was associated with risk of harm rather than the complexity of the decision.

6. Reference Guide to Consent for Examination or Treatment, Department of Health; Chapter 1 (www.doh.gov.uk/consent). BMA and the Law Society, Assessment of mental capacity: guidance for doctors and lawyers, 1995 (www.bma.org.uk).
7. Per Lord Bridge in *Re F*, 1990, 2 AC at 5. The courts have jurisdiction only to rule on the *legality* of a proposed treatment so that any treatment will not be considered and assault. The courts cannot and do not give consent on behalf of the patient. The *parens patria* jurisdiction of the courts which effectively permitted incompetent adults to become wards of the court (thereby allowing the courts to provide consent) was ended in 1960.
8. *Re F or F v West Berkshire Health Authority*, 1989, 2 All ER 545.
9. *Bolam v Friern Hospital Management Committee*, 1957, 2 All ER 118. See chapter on medical negligence *infra*.
10. *Re MB, supra*.
11. Adults with Incapacity (Scotland) Act 2000.
12. *F v West Berkshire Health Authority*, 1989, 2 All ER 545. Per Lord Goff at 566.
13. Dyer C. *Brit Med J*, 1997, 315:832. A gynaecologist was censured by the GMC for removing ovaries without consent during a hysterectomy (for which there was consent). An example also of exceeding consent.
14. Interventions ranging from nasogastic feeding of an anorexic patient Re KB (adult: medical treatment of mental patient), 1994, 19 BMLR 144. To a Caesarean section; *Tameside & Glossop Acute Services Trust v CH*, 1996, 1 Fam LR. 762.
15. Mental Health Act 1983, Department of Health and Welsh Office, Codes of Practice: Mental Health Act 1983 (1999) The Stationary Office, London. S58 sets out additional safeguards that apply to ECT and medication after three months has elapsed since first administration of the medication. S57 provides safeguards in respect of surgery to alleviate a mental illness. S62 MHA allows for S57 and S58 to be overridden in the case of an emergency.
16. *Re C (Adult: Refusal of Medical Treatment)*, 1994, 1 All ER 819.
17. *St George's Healthcare Trust v S*, 1998, 3 All ER 673.
18. Maclean AR. Caesarean sections, competence and the illusion of autonomy, 1999, 1 Web JCLI.
19. Seeking patients' consent; the ethical considerations, GMC 1998. (www.gmc-uk.org).
20. *Airdale NHS Trust v Bland*, 1993, 1 All ER 821.
21. *National Health Service Trust v D and Others*, 2000, 55 BMLR 19.
22. Now incorporated into UK domestic law by the Human Rights Act 1998.
23. The principle cases have involved cessation of medical treatment in respect of patients kept alive by artificial means. In Re Quinlan, 1976, NJSC, *Brophy v New England Sinai Hospital*.
24. The Children Act 1989 describes minors as being someone who had not reached their 18th birthday. For convenience the groups are commonly divided into young persons of 16 and 17 years of age and children under the age of 16.
25. Age of Majority Act (Northern Ireland) 1969, Age of Capacity (Scotland) Act 1991.
26. MDU Consent to Medical Treatment, 1996.
27. *Gillick v West Norfolk and Wisbech AHA*, 1986, 3 AC 112. The case related to the legality of GP's providing contraceptive advise to under 16s but the principles

enunciated now provide general guidance in respect of all forms of treatment involving the under 16s.

28. *Ibid.* per Lord Fraser. Though Lord Scarman made no such best interest requirement suggesting that a competent child's refusal should be equated with an adult's right to refuse and could not be overridden.

29. Age of Legal Capacity (Scotland) Act 1991, S2(4).

30. *Re R (A minor: wardship consent to medical treatment)*, 1991, 4 All ER 177.

31. 1992, 4 All ER 627.

32. *Re L (A minor)*, 1998, 51 BMLR.

33. *Re C*, 1997, 40 BMLR 32.

34. *Sidaway v Bethlem Royal Hospital Governors and Others*, All ER 1985, 1.

35. *Chatterton v Gerson*, 1981, 1 All ER 257.

36. *Canterbury v Spence*, 1972, 464 F 2d 772 in the USA, *Reibl v Hughes*, 1980, 114 DLR (3d) 1 in Canada, and *Rogers v Whitaker*, 1992, 67 AWR 47 in Australia.

37. *Canterbury v Spence*, 1972, 464 F 2d 772 at 787.

38. *Rogers v Whittaker, ibid.*

39. *Pearce v United Bristol Healthcare NHS Trust*, 1999, 48 BMLR 118.

40. *Bolitho v City and Hackney Health Authority*, 1997, 39 BMLR 1.

41. See www.bma.org.uk, www.gmc-uk.org (seehug patients consent: the ethical considerations, GMC.

42. Except the Human Fertilisation and Embryology Act 1990 where written consent in a legal requirement for the storage and use of gametes (www.hfea.gov.uk).

6

Professional bodies and discipline

Jason Payne-James and Julie Smith

INTRODUCTION

This chapter outlines the broad principles of health professional regulation within the UK. The regulation of standards of different healthcare professionals varies widely, and there are a number of specific 'professional regulators' responsible for several professions. These are listed in Table 6.1. Other organisations are involved in the monitoring and assessment of standards and these are listed in Table 6.2. Some professions have disciplinary procedures that are controlled by statute and others by codes of practice or guidelines set by bodies established for that purpose alone, or by bodies supervising or giving advice on a whole range

Table 6.1 Professional regulators.
Health Professions Council
Dental Practice Board
General Chiropractic Council
General Dental Council
General Medical Council
General Optical Council
General Osteopathic Council
Royal Pharmaceutical Society of Great Britain
Nursing & Midwifery Council

Table 6.2 Quality and Standards.
Audit Commission
Clinical Standards Board for Scotland
National Audit Office
National Care Standards Commission
The Health Quality Service

of issues, such as negotiating for pay and conditions, or supervising under-graduate and postgraduate education.

The amount of self-regulation of the professions has been an area of great concern although successive governments have supported the concept that it is a satisfactory means of control when backed by statute and financially independent of the state. The majority of regulatory bodies have a role in setting or defining standards of practise and pro-vide the means by which practitioners who have deemed to have failed to achieve such standards can be disciplined. The body will thus be the key source of accountability for a practitioner within their profession. Sanctions vary dependant on the regulating body and may, for example, allow for the removal of a practitioner from a register (thereby possibly depriving them of their livelihood) or for the supervision of that practi-tioner when working, or make requirements for training. Some profes-sions have been organised as individuals, others as groups.

Osteopathy is one of the professions that has developed on its own via statute. The Osteopaths Act 1993 created the General Osteopathic Council and since 9 May 2000, the title 'Osteopath' is protected by law. It is a criminal offence, liable to prosecution, for anyone to claim to be any kind of osteopath unless registered with the General Osteopathic Council.[1] The Health Professions Council (HPC)[2] was set up to safe-guard the health and well-being of patients using the services of the spe-cific professions it regulates (see Table 6.3) and to ensure that the public has access to, and are treated by health professionals who are qualified

Table 6.3 Number of registrants with HPC (on 1 April 2003).	
Profession	Registrants
Art therapists	1 992
Chiropodists/podiatrists	9 013
Clinical scientists	3 408
Dietitians	5 782
Medical laboratory technicians	21 895
Occupational therapists	24 576
Orthoptists	1 328
Prosthetists and orthotists	786
Paramedics	9 334
Physiotherapists	35 643
Radiographers	21 484
Speech and language therapists	8 900
Total	**144 141**

and competent. The HPC replaced the old Council for Professions Supplementary to Medicine (CPSM), created by the Professions Supplementary to Medicine Act 1960 and was itself established by the Health Professions Order 2001. The Council of the HPC is responsible for developing strategies and policies and consists of 24 members (made up of one representative from each of the professions regulated and 12 lay members) and a president. There are 12 alternate professional members who attend Council and Committee meetings in the absence of the 12 representatives. Four statutory committees have been set up to deal with conduct and competence, the health of professionals registered with HPC, investigating complaints and the establishment and monitoring of training and education standards. All committees are chaired by a member of the Council and they make recommendations and decisions in consultation with the Council.

The roles and functions of the General Medical Council (GMC) – for doctors, nurses and the Nursing & Midwifery Council (NMC) – will now be considered in detail as examples to illustrate the working of professional regulatory bodies.

GMC

The GMC was first established by statute by the Medical Act 1858 and consisted of a membership of 24, all of whom were medically qualified and who represented the Royal Colleges, the Universities, and the Privy Council. This Act was intended in part to enable 'persons requiring medical aid ... to distinguish qualified from unqualified practitioners'. In order to achieve this a register was created. Subsequent Medical Acts – the most recent being the Medical Act 1983 – which consolidated previous Acts, expanded the role and workload of the GMC. In addition its activities have – as a result of a number of high profile cases involving doctors – come under unprecedented external scrutiny and critical examination from within the profession itself. Further recent legislation discussed below has been produced in part as a result of these criticisms and has changed the ways in which the GMC scrutinises a doctor's 'fitness-to-practice'. The GMC's role is limited to the powers and duties conferred by statute. It is not a general complaints body and can only act where there is evidence that a doctor may not be fit to practise. As such its actions may be subject to public law challenge by the route of judicial review. The GMC explains its current role in the following terms:[3]

> Protecting the public: We have strong and effective legal powers designed to maintain the standards the public have a right to expect of doctors.

We are not here to protect the medical profession – their interests are protected by others. Our job is to protect patients.

The public trust doctors to set and monitor their own professional standards. In return doctors must give their patients high-quality medical care. Where any doctor fails to meet those standards, we act to protect patients from harm, if necessary, by striking the doctor off the register and removing their right to practise medicine.

We are a charity whose purpose is the protection, promotion and maintenance of the health and safety of the community

The majority of the GMC's income is derived from the registration of new members and from the annual retention fees of existing members.

Structure and functions of the GMC

Until 2003, the GMC was a vast structure of 104 members, 54 medically qualified doctors who were elected by the doctors on the register, 25 members of the public nominated by the Privy Council and 25 doctors appointed by educational bodies – the universities, medical royal colleges and faculties. Privy Council nominees are not medically qualified and their role is to speak for the public, enabling the GMC to act as a focus for debate between doctors and patients.

In December 2002, the Privy Council agreed new legislation which allowed the most comprehensive and wide ranging reform of professional regulation since the establishment of the GMC in 1858. The three main elements to the proposals are: constitutional reform by reducing the size of the Council from 104 to 35 and increasing lay membership from 25% to 40%; reform of 'fitness-to-practice' procedures and how complaints about doctors are dealt with; and reform of registration procedures – with the introduction of revalidation – a regular demonstration by doctors that they meet standards required for continued registration. The current powers were set out in the Medical Act 1983 and subsequently amended by various other primary and secondary legislation. The new changes are set out in the Medical Act 1983 (Amendment Order) 2002. The reformed Council met for the first time in July 2003 after elections earlier in 2003, and consists of 19 elected medical members, 14 lay members nominated by the Privy Council and two medical members appointed by the Council of Heads of Medical Schools and the Academy of Medical Royal Colleges.

Registration

The GMC is a body which sets standards for undergraduate pre-registration and postgraduate medical education. Doctors must be

Table 6.4 Examples of statutes with defined roles/functions for medical practitioners.

Abortion Act 1967
Access to Medical Records Act 1990
Air Force Act 1955
Armed Forces Act 1981
Army Act 1955
Births & Death Registration Act 1953
Cancer Act 1939
Children Act 1989
Children & Young Persons Act 1969
Chiropractors Act 1994
Courts-Martial (Appeals) Act 1968
Crime (Sentences) Act 1997
Crime & Disorder Act 1998
Criminal Appeal Act 1968
Criminal Justice Act 1967
Local Government Finance Act 1992
Magistrates' Courts Act 1980
Marriage Act 1949
Medicines Act 1968
Mental Health Act 1983
Misuse of Drugs Act 1971
National Health Service & Community Care Act 1990
Opticians Act 1989
Public Health (Control of Disease) Act 1984

registered with the GMC to practise medicine in the UK. To register with the GMC, they must have a recognised medical qualification. Currently new requirements are being introduced that all doctors must demonstrate their continuing fitness to practise in order to remain registered – a process called revalidation. The medical register shows who is properly qualified to practise medicine in the UK. About 200,000 doctors are registered. Registration confers certain privileges allowing doctors to undertake certain procedures or functions. The full list is published on the GMC website.[4] Examples of statutes which specifically refer to medical practitioners as having a role or function are given in Table 6.4. The type of work that requires doctors to be registered includes: employment in the National Health Service (NHS); prescribing certain drugs; issuing medical certificates required for statutory purposes.

Doctors wishing to work in private practice (non-NHS appointments) in the UK must also register with the GMC because the major private health hospitals and insurers only recognise registered doctors. The process for gaining registration is generally dependant on the nationality of the applicant and the country where the primary medical qualification was obtained. There are a number of main groups of doctors for the purposes of registration. These are: doctors qualifying from a UK medical school are eligible for provisional and full registration; doctors qualifying in another European Economic Area (EEA) Member State and who are nationals of an EEA Member State (or non-EEA nationals with European Community (EC) rights) are eligible for full registration (they are also eligible to apply for provisional registration if their medical education includes a period of postgraduate clinical training); doctors qualifying in Australia, Hong Kong, Malaysia, New Zealand, Singapore, South Africa, and the West Indies may be eligible for provisional and full registration; doctors who qualify in other countries not listed above may be eligible for limited and full registration and include non-EEA nationals who do not benefit under EC law who have qualified in another EEA Member State. Finally, EEA nationals (and non-EEA nationals with EC rights) who qualify in other countries not listed above may be eligible for provisional or full registration if they have practised medicine in another EEA Member State.

Full registration is required for unsupervised medical practise in the NHS or private practice in the UK. Specialist registration may be required for a consultant post within the NHS. Provisional registration allows newly qualified doctors to undertake the general clinical training needed for full registration. A provisionally registered doctor is entitled to work only in resident junior house officer posts in hospitals or institutions. The period of pre-registration is normally one year. Limited registration requires an appropriate primary qualification. Applicants for limited registration must provide evidence of their current capability for practise in the UK either by passing the Professional Linguistic Assessment Board (PLAB) test or by providing other evidence. Limited registration is only for supervised employment in training posts in the NHS for a maximum of five years.

The GMC also maintains the Specialist Register. Since 1 January 1997 it has been a legal requirement that to hold a consultant post (other than a locum consultant appointment) in a medical or surgical specialty in the NHS a doctor must be included in the Specialist Register. Exceptions are doctors who held a consultant post (other than a locum consultant post) in oral and maxillofacial surgery in the NHS immediately before 1 January 1997.

The GMC emphasises that registration carries both privileges and responsibilities. The duties of a doctor, which the GMC describes as the

Table 6.5 Duties of a doctor.

As a doctor one must:

- make the care of their patient their first concern
- treat every patient politely and considerately
- respect patients' dignity and privacy
- listen to patients and respect their views
- give patients information in a way they can understand
- respect the rights of patients to be fully involved in decisions about their care
- keep their professional knowledge and skills up to date
- recognise the limits of their professional competence
- be honest and trustworthy
- respect and protect confidential information
- make sure that their personal beliefs do not prejudice their patients' care
- act quickly to protect patients from risk if they have good reason to believe that they or a colleague may not be fit to practise
- avoid abusing their position as a doctor and
- work with colleagues in the ways that best serve patients' interests

'contract between doctor and patient which is at the heart of medicine' are listed in Table 6.5. The GMC provides specific guidance in a wide range of medical areas including confidentiality,[5] research,[6] withholding and withdrawing life-prolonging treatments,[7] serious communicable diseases,[8] and consent.[9] Such guidance describes the principles of good medical practice and standards of competence, care and conduct expected of doctors in all aspects of their professional work. Serious or persistent failures to meet these standards may put a doctor's registration at risk.

Fitness-to-practice procedures

The GMC's fitness-to-practice procedures and powers are linked to licensing doctors and maintaining the medical register. A doctor's registration can be restricted or removed if one of the fitness-to-practice committees decides that this is necessary. The GMC can take action against doctors if the doctor has been convicted of a criminal offence; if there is evidence of conduct that appears to be so serious that it is likely to call into question the doctor's fitness to continue in medical practise (serious professional misconduct, SPM); if there is evidence of a repeated departure from good professional practice, whether or not it is covered by

Table 6.6 Examples of why the GMC may need to intervene.

Serious or repeated mistakes in carrying out medical procedures or in
    diagnosis, for example incorrect dosages on prescriptions, prescribing
    inappropriate drugs
Failure to examine patients properly or respond reasonably to patient
    needs
Fraud or dishonesty in financial matters or in dealings with patients or
    research
Serious breaches of a patient's confidentiality
Treating patients without making sure that they know what is involved
    and agree to it
Making sexual advances towards patients
Misusing alcohol or drugs

specific GMC guidance, sufficiently serious to call into question a doctor's
registration (seriously deficient performance); or if there is evidence
that a doctor is not fit to practise medicine because of the state of his or
her health. There are certain rules which the fitness-to-practice committees are bound by. These rules have recently been streamlined by the
GMC (Fitness to Practice Committees) (Amendment) Rules Order of
Council 2002. Table 6.6 illustrates examples of cases where the GMC
may need to intervene. Complaints may arise from a variety of sources
including patients, fellow doctors, other healthcare professionals, the
police, government departments, NHS authorities and others who employ
doctors. Any doctor whose 'fitness-to-practice' is questioned should seek
advice from their own medical defence organisation (MDO).

In the event of a complaint the first stage is for one of the GMC's
caseworkers to assess whether concerns should be investigated further.
If it is decided that a case does need to be considered further under one
of the GMC's procedures, the next step will be to obtain all relevant
information required to assess the case properly and may involve some
or all of the following – a written account of the complaint; copies of any
relevant medical records or reports; copies of any relevant correspondence will be required if complaints have been made directly to the doctor or to another organisation. Before a formal decision on a case can be
taken, the doctor concerned will be given an opportunity to comment
on the allegations. Once all the evidence is available, the case will be
considered by one or more council members appointed as 'screeners'.
Their role is to consider whether a case raises concerns about a doctor
which are so serious that they need to be referred to the next stage of

the GMC's fitness-to-practice procedures; and if so which of the procedures would be the best way of examining the concerns. All cases will initially be reviewed by a medical member. If the medical member decides that no action is required the case will not be closed without the agreement of a second, lay member. If either the medical member or the lay member decides that the case does raise serious concerns it will be placed under one (or more) of the following procedures: conduct, performance, or health. If both agree that there is no need for any further action against the doctor, the GMC will write to the complainant and to the doctor explaining the decision. It is not normally possible to appeal against this decision. The GMC aims to be able to take a screening decision within six months of receiving a complaint. If there is evidence that the doctor poses an immediate risk to patients the GMC will ensure that the case is dealt with quickly, and will ask the Interim Orders Committee (*vide infra*) to decide whether the doctor should be suspended or have conditions imposed on his registration while enquiries continue.

Conduct procedures

The GMC's conduct procedures consider allegations of SPM, and deal with doctors convicted of criminal offences (excluding minor motoring offences). Conduct procedures are governed by Schedule 4 of the Medical Act 1983 and the amended GMC Preliminary Proceedings Committee and Professional Conduct Committee (Procedure) Rules 1988. The Preliminary Procedure Committee (PPC) is a panel of medical and lay members. The Committee meets in private to decide whether a case should be referred to the Professional Conduct Committee (PCC) for a full formal inquiry in public. Criminal cases involving custodial sentences can be fast-tracked to a full hearing of the PCC. If the PPC decides that there is no need to refer the case to the PCC they may still provide the doctor with advice about their future conduct. The rules which govern the GMC's procedures do not allow for an appeal against a PPC decision. If either screener decides that a case raises a possible issue of SPM, the GMC will write formally to the doctor setting out the allegations against him. The doctor then has a further chance to comment before the case is considered by the PPC. The GMC will ask the doctor if he agrees to these comments being disclosed to the complainant.

The PCC is the final stage of the GMC's conduct procedures. The inquiries are conducted in public and the doctor has a chance to respond in person to the allegations. Before the PCC meets to consider a case, the GMC's solicitors will prepare the case by arranging for witness statements, expert reports and any other information needed to bring the case against the doctor. The complainant and other witnesses will need to give evidence under oath, with questioning from the panel hearing the case, and lawyers representing both sides. If a doctor is found guilty of SPM the PCC can: erase the doctor from the register; suspend the doctor's registration; impose conditions on the doctor's registration; or give the doctor a warning. If the PCC finds that the doctor is not guilty of SPM it may decide to take no action against the doctor or may issue advice about future conduct. The PCC's decision to impose conditions on registration, suspend or strike off a doctor takes effect in about 28 days after it is announced. If the Committee orders that a doctor is suspended or struck off, and believe that others could be put at risk, or that it would be in the doctors' interests to stop medical work at once, suspension of registration can be imposed immediately. Application to the High Court can be made to have that order lifted. There are 28 days to appeal to the Judicial Committee of the Privy Council against the decision to suspend registration or impose conditions. These appeal procedures apply for all fitness-to-practice decisions.

Performance procedures

The GMC's performance procedures assess doctors whose performance appears to be seriously deficient. Performance procedures are governed by Schedule 4 of the Medical Act 1983 and the amended GMC (Professional Performance) Rules 1997. If the GMC receives information that suggests a doctor may be performing poorly they will first establish whether there is a case to answer – there is initial consideration by a screener. The screener does not have to notify the doctor at this stage. If the screener considers there is a case, the GMC will invite the doctor to undergo an assessment of their skills and knowledge – a performance assessment. If the doctor refuses to participate or undergo an assessment they will be referred to the Assessment Referral Committee (ARC). The ARC has power to direct the doctor to undergo an assessment within a fixed period of time. A complainant has the opportunity to be heard at the ARC meeting. The assessment is carried out by a team of trained assessors. The assessment team will normally include two doctors from the relevant specialty and a member of the public. The assessment will cover the doctor's attitudes, knowledge, clinical and communications skills, and clinical records and audit results. After the assessment the team will report to the case co-ordinator, a medical member of the Council who supervises the performance cases. The case co-ordinator will decide on the next step. This may be: to take no further action if the assessment has revealed no serious performance problems; to ask that the doctor takes action to improve his performance (if the problems have been identified but they pose no risk to patients); to refer the doctor to the Committee of Professional Performance (CPP) if serious problems have been identified. The CPP may, if necessary, suspend or place conditions on the doctor's registration. After two years, registration may be suspended indefinitely. Complainants are usually unlikely to be required in person at a hearing unless they express a wish to attend.

Health procedures

Health procedures can be utilised if a doctor is attempting to practise despite being seriously affected by ill health. The GMC – in addition to protecting patients – will also encourage the doctor to seek appropriate treatment with a view to returning to work if possible. The most serious cases are reported to the Health Committee (HC), which can suspend or place conditions on the doctor's registration. Procedures are governed by Schedule 4 of the Medical Act 1983 and the amended GMC Health Committee (Procedure) Rules 1987. The central feature of the health procedures is a medical assessment by experts. Any issues raising questions about health are referred to a 'health screener' – a GMC member who is a psychiatrist. The health screener decides whether patients are being put at risk, and considers whether there is enough evidence to suggest that the ability to practise may be seriously impaired by a physical or mental condition. The health screener will also consider whether the problem has been, or could be, put right by local action. The health screener may decide not to get involved if they believe that local measures, which are already being taken, will prevent harm to patients. If the health screener decides on further action, examination will be proposed by at least two medical examiners chosen by the GMC – but who are not GMC members. Psychiatric issues including addiction are the most common reasons for referral and thus the examiners are likely to be consultant psychiatrists. Examinations by other specialists are arranged as necessary – including submission of 'medical evidence' by the doctor being examined. After examination reports are made about the state of health and ability to practise, if it is decided that treatment is required, recommendations will be made about medical supervision and support advised which might be limitations, including avoiding single-handed practice; practising only if supervised; or not practising medicine at all.

If the reports state that the doctor is fit for medical work, the health screener will close the case. If it is believed ability to practise is seriously impaired by a medical condition, the screener will ask the doctor to accept recommendations for medical supervision and for restrictions on medical work. Once agreement has been reached about medical supervision, the health screener will choose a doctor to supervise and to arrange necessary treatment. Limitations on medical work will reduce as health improves. Once the screener decides the doctor can practise medicine again without restriction, there will be further reports from the medical supervisor and the GMC will not be further involved.

In most cases, doctors under the health procedures co-operate, however the HC will become involved if the doctor: does not agree to be medically examined; refuses to accept recommendations for medical supervision or limitations on medical work; does not keep to the agreement to follow the recommendations they have accepted; or their state of health deteriorates further.

There are nine members of the HC which meets in private and adopts legal rules of procedure. Seven are medical members and two are lay (non-medical) members. All the HC members are GMC members. At the hearing, the Committee receives advice from two specialist medical assessors selected from lists put forward by the royal colleges and others. A legal assessor is present to advise on points of law. The main evidence at the hearings is the written medical reports. If the Committee wants more evidence before they make a decision, they may postpone the hearing for a set period so they can find that evidence. Alternatively, they may adjourn the hearing if the doctor agrees to have medical treatment and to limit professional work. The Committee must decide whether ability to practise is seriously impaired by a health problem. If it is, they may suspend registration for up to 12 months; or put conditions on registration for up to three years. The Committee will consider the case again at the end of the period of suspension or when the conditions are due to be reviewed – and another medical examination will generally be undertaken before the hearing. The Committee will decide whether there is any risk to patients on the basis of the evidence, including up-to-date reports from the medical supervisor. If they then decide to close the case, the doctor can return to medical work, without any restrictions. If the case is kept under review, further conditions can be imposed, or registration suspended for up to a year at a time. If the Committee have suspended registration for two years, registration can then be suspended indefinitely. There would then be no need for further hearings unless requested by the doctor.

Interim Orders Committee

The GMC has powers to either suspend or place conditions on a doctor's registration at any stage in their procedures. This can be done when the doctor may be a risk to patients; when the doctor may be a risk to himself;

when it is in the public interest. The Interim Orders Committee's role is to consider the application of interim measures on a doctor's registration while fitness-to-practice procedures continue. This is a very severe sanction that is only applied when there is evidence of a clear need to act immediately to suspend or restrict a doctor.

Other relevant bodies

The National Clinical Assessment Authority (NCAA) was set up by the government to deal with under-performing doctors and aims to reduce the number and length of suspensions.[10] The NCAA is a special health authority established on 1 April 2001. The NCAA is an example of the government's and medical profession's shared commitment to supporting the principles of best practise, clear standards, high quality, and patient safety. The GMC has agreements (Memoranda of Understanding) with the NCAA, Commission for Health Improvement (CHI), and the National Care Standards Commission to ensure they work together effectively to protect patients. The aim of the NCAA is to provide a support service to NHS primary care, hospital and community trusts, the Prison Health Service and the Defence Medical Services when they are faced with concerns over the performance of an individual doctor. In order to help doctors in difficulty, the NCAA provides advice, takes referrals and carries out targeted assessments where necessary. The NCAA's assessment involves trained medical and lay assessors. Once an objective assessment has been carried out, the NCAA will advise on the appropriate course of action. The NCAA does not take over the role of an employer, nor will it function as a regulator. The NCAA is established as an advisory body, and the NHS employer organisation remains responsible for resolving the problem once the NCAA has produced its assessment.

Appraisal and revalidation

Appraisal has been introduced by the Department of Health in England for doctors working in the NHS. The aim is to give doctors regular feedback on past performance and continuing progress and to identify education and development needs – it is part of a doctor's career development. At the same time as appraisal was being developed, the GMC made proposals to licence and revalidate all registered doctors. The aims of appraisal are shown in Table 6.7.

Currently in the UK, the following are subject to appraisal schemes: consultants, including clinical academic consultants and public health consultants; non-consultant career grade doctors, including staff grades,

Table 6.7 Aims of appraisal.

To set out personal and professional development needs, career paths, and goals

To agree plans for them to be met

To review the doctor's performance

To consider the doctor's contribution to the quality and improvement of local healthcare services

To optimise the use of skills and resources in achieving the delivery of high-quality care

To offer an opportunity for doctors to discuss and seek support for their participation in activities

To identify the need for adequate resources to enable service objectives to be met

associate specialists, clinical assistants, hospital practitioners, community and senior medical officers, trust doctors and others on local contracts; GP principals. Appraisal for other groups of doctors will be introduced in due course. Details of appraisal may be found at www.appraisaluk.info.

For NHS doctors, appraisal will also be the method for gathering revalidation evidence. All doctors must have a licence to practice to treat patients or prescribe for them. Every five years each doctor who wants to remain in practice must present evidence to the GMC that they are competent in their field of practise and have kept up to date. This will allow the doctor's licence to practise to be renewed.

To simplify matters the Department of Health and the GMC agreed that a single set of documentation would be used for appraisal and revalidation. For doctors within managed organisations, five sets of completed annual appraisal forms can be submitted to the GMC as evidence to support revalidation. Alternatively, the evidence gathered for the appraisal process could also be submitted to the GMC as evidence to support revalidation.

Although appraisal is designed to help doctors identify development needs and produce personal development plans, rather than assess performance, evidence of participation will confirm that the doctor is discussing the quality of his or her own work and keeping up to date. This is strongly supportive of fitness and overall qualification to practise medicine.

The current status of revalidation is as follows. If a doctor in the future wishes to continue to practise (including prescribing and signing statutory certificates), a licence to practise will be required. The GMC will grant doctors a licence to practise by the end of 2004, unless they tell the GMC they don't want one. If a doctor is not on the register by the end of 2004, they will get a licence automatically when they are registered. To maintain a licence to practise doctors must take part in revalidation when requested by the GMC. It is intended that the GMC will start to invite doctors for revalidation in Spring 2005, but as yet it is unknown when the first revalidation will be. During 2004 doctors will be asked to tell the GMC if they do not want a licence to practise. Otherwise, if they are on the register – no matter what type of registration – they will be granted a licence to practise by the end of 2004. This will mean that the GMC thinks the doctor is properly qualified, and that they have agreed to take part in periodic revalidation. By 1 January 2005, by law, a doctor will not be able to practise without a licence.

To keep a licence to practise, the GMC will ask each doctor, normally once every five years, to show them that they have been practising medicine in line with the standards set out in the publication Good Medical Practice.[11] Revalidation is the combination of the doctor doing this, and the GMC confirming that their licence will continue. Doctors will need to be able to show the GMC that they have followed the standards which are relevant to their specialty and their practice. It is the doctor's own responsibility, not that of others. The doctor must decide how to show the GMC that they have followed these standards. The two main ways in which this can be done, and the GMC will either accept or, if it helps a combination of the two through which most doctors will be able to use, is the appraisal route. The second is the independent route in which the doctor will have to show that they are adopting the standards of Good Medical Practice[11] within their professional practice and undertaking appropriate continuing medical education or professional development.

The GMC will tell doctors the result of their own revalidation as soon as they can. The licence will, of course, remain valid until they have made the final decision about the revalidation. The possible outcomes are: revalidation – the licence to practise will remain valid; insufficient information – the GMC cannot revalidate the doctor because they have not given them enough information and the doctor will be asked to provide additional information needed, and then the case will be reconsidered; and inadequate information – when the GMC is not persuaded by the information the doctor has provided, including the additional information that was asked for, that they should be revalidated. The GMC will only withdraw a licence if: the doctor tells them they no longer want it; the doctor does not pay the appropriate fee; the doctor does not take part in the revalidation process when they ask them to, or a fitness-to-practice panel directs that the doctor's registration should be suspended or erased. A doctor will have the right of appeal against any decision to withdraw, or refuse to restore their licence to practise. Further and regularly updated information on revalidation is located at www.revalidationuk.info. It is likely that both appraisal and revalidation will continue to modify, change, and evolve substantially in the next few years.

NMC (FORMERLY UKCC)

The NMC succeeded the UKCC on the 1 April 2002. Its powers are set out in the Nursing & Midwifery Order 2001.[12] The core function of the NMC is to 'establish and improve standards of nursing, midwifery, and health visiting care in order to serve and protect the public'[13] and as such keeps a register of all practitioners. All healthcare professionals in the field of nursing are required to re-register their intention to practice every three years and must produce evidence of current practice and professional development in the preceding five years to retain their registration.

Other core functions of the NMC include: responsibility for assuring quality in nursing, health visiting, and midwifery education; provision of an advisory service and to consider allegations of misconduct or unfitness to practise due to ill health. The NMC has the power to confer, remove, or suspend practitioners from the register.

The Council is made up of 35 members – 12 registrant members, 12 alternative registrant members and 11 lay members. The registrant members consist of equal numbers of nurses, health visitors, and midwives, the lay membership is made up of people from education, employment, and consumer groups. There is a President and Vice President.

The NMC issues a Code of Conduct for practitioners, all members of the nursing profession are required to practice within the Code and are personally accountable for their practice (either action or omission) regardless of direction or advice from another professional.

Professional conduct

The current Code of Conduct was published in April 2002 and came into effect on 1 June 2002. It is a clear and concise document that emphasises a practitioner's personal accountability for their practice and continuing professional development.

Misconduct

The NMC only deals with misconduct that, if proven, would be serious enough to justify removal of the practitioner from the register. The purpose of removal is to protect the public, not punish the practitioner. On this basis, conduct that results in dismissal from employment would not necessarily lead to removal from the register. Thus there are a number of similarities to GMC processes.

Allegations that would justify removal from the register must be capable of proof. The PCC applies the criminal standard of proof to the evidence it receives and has to be 'satisfied beyond reasonable doubt' that the allegation is proven. The secondary consideration of professional misconduct is subsequently addressed.

A PPC considers whether a case of alleged misconduct should be referred to a hearing by the PCC. The hearing is held in public and the practitioner may be legally represented.

There is no automatic list of offences that lead to removal from the register. Types of misconduct that may result in removal include, physical or verbal abuse of patients, failure to keep proper records, failure to care for patients properly, and theft from patients.

A complaint alleging misconduct can be made by anyone and should be sent in writing to the NMC.

Fitness to practise

The NMC only deals with cases where a practitioners' condition seriously impairs their fitness to practise. Once again the primary purpose of suspension or removal from the register is to protect the public. A practitioner who voluntarily stops working when unable to practice safely, through ill health is not a risk to the public and therefore the NMC does not need to make a decision.

The HC when satisfied that a practitioner is unfit to practice is empowered to remove or suspend a practitioner from the register. A report to the NMC concerning fitness to practise must be made in the form of a statutory declaration. This is prepared by the NMC's solicitors and a copy is sent to the practitioner. HC hearings are held in private. Conditions that may seriously impair fitness to practise include: drug and/or alcohol dependence; untreated serious mental illness; and personality disorder.

Interim suspension

In exceptional cases either in misconduct or unfitness, the NMC can suspend a practitioners' registration prior to a hearing by the appropriate committee. This will occur where the PPC considers there is evidence that constitutes a continuing serious risk either to the public or to the practitioner.

CLINICAL GOVERNANCE

Reporting of major failures in the NHS in recent years, such as the Bristol, Shipman, and Allitt enquiries, has highlighted the need for comprehensive risk management and robust reporting mechanisms throughout the NHS. To achieve better monitoring and safer clinical practise, the concept of clinical governance has been formalised into a framework. Clinical governance can be defined as 'a framework through which NHS organisations are accountable for continuously improving the quality of their services and safeguarding high standards of care by creating an environment in which excellence in clinical care will flourish'.[14]

Emphasis is now placed on integrated quality improvement systems incorporating clinical audit, risk management, evidence-based practise, adverse incident reporting and a whole range of other processes that are designed to identify and disseminate areas of good practise and areas where improvements in patient care and safety can be made. While labelled as 'clinical governance' the term covers any system or process within the NHS that has a direct impact on the quality of patient care, therefore management decisions can constitute a clinical governance issue and be reportable as such.

An open, honest, fair blame culture is the desired result of the clinical governance framework throughout the NHS where mistakes were made, can be analysed openly and lessons can be learnt to protect patients and support practitioners.

The principles of clinical governance apply to all those who provide or manage patient care services in the NHS and are inextricably linked to those underpinning professional self-regulation. Both are the business of every registered practitioner and all have a responsibility to themselves, their colleagues and their patients to contribute and respond to the clinical governance framework of their organisation. It is worth noting when identifying a concern about a colleagues' practise or a management system/process the first question asked by the CHI will be 'and what did you do about it?'.

REFERENCES

1. www.osteopathy.org.uk.
2. www.hpc-uk.org.
3. www.gmc-uk.org.
4. www.gmc-uk.org/register/p&o.

5. General Medical Council. *Confidentiality: Protecting and Providing Information*, GMC, 2000.
6. General Medical Council. *Research: The Role and Responsibilities of Doctors*, GMC, 2002.
7. General Medical Council. *Withholding and Withdrawing Life-Prolonging Treatments: Good Practice in Decision-Making*, GMC, 2002.
8. General Medical Council. *Serious Communicable Diseases*, GMC, 1997.
9. General Medical Council. *Seeking Patients Consent: The Ethical Considerations*, GMC, 1998.
10. www.ncaa.nhs.uk.
11. General Medical Council. *Good Medical Practice*, GMC, 2001.
12. www.hmso.gov.uk (Nursing and Midwifery Order, Statutory Instrument 2002/253).
13. www.nmc-uk.org (What the NMC does).
14. A First Class Service. *Quality in the new NHS*. Department of Health, 1998.

7

Complaints in the National Health Service

George Fernie

INTRODUCTION

While there are now a considerable variety of routes of accountability that a member of the medical profession may be subject to, the most common almost certainly continues to be the National Health Service (NHS) Complaints Procedure given that the majority of consultations in the UK will take place in this context.

There remains confusion amongst doctors as to what constitutes a claim as opposed to a complaint. At its most simplistic, a claim is where there has been a breach of the duty of care owed resulting in harm to that individual whose intention is to obtain financial recompense, as the doctor has allegedly not provided the standard of care provided as defined by case law. In contrast, a complaint has been described by the Citizen's Charter Complaints Task Force as '*an expression of dissatisfaction requiring a response*'. The Citizen's Charter Task Force was created by the Conservative Government of that time and published a report in June 1995 on the handling of complaints in the public sector.

It is not unknown for an adverse incident to initially be dealt with through one of these routes but ultimately to lead to the civil courts in an attempt to obtain restitution. It may be that a doctor first answers through the NHS Complaints Procedure, goes to the health service commissioner by route of appeal, is reported to the General Medical Council (GMC), may even end up in the criminal courts and is eventually sued by way of a claim in the system known as tort in England and delict in Scotland. The Health Service Ombudsman investigates complaints about the National Health Service. There is a necessity that prior to asking the Ombudsman to look into a complaint this must first be taken up locally with the body that is being complained about. Not only is the Ombudsman (Health Service Commissioner) completely independent of the NHS and the Government but there is no charge for the Ombudsman's service although the Ombudsman does have to investigate the complaint.

71

Whichever side of the border a civil claim begins, the ultimate court of appeal in the UK is the House of Lords and while academics may try and argue on the distinguishing features of cases such as Hunter v Hanley[1] or Bolam v Friern,[2] subsequent case law modifying these principles as found in Bolitho has almost certainly affected the way we practise throughout the UK albeit the new Civil Procedure Rules emanating from the Woolf reforms only apply in England and Wales.

With the advent of the new NHS Complaints Procedure, most medical defence organisations (MDOs) found an increase of at least 50% in such workload both in the GP sector which makes up around ⅔ of their cases and similarly with hospital patients.[3]

The changes that took place in all the professions during previous governments with an increasing emphasis on accountability coupled to ready access to clinical records through various statutes culminating in the Data Protection Act 1988 allowed a patient to determine whether or not they had received the required level of care.

The Patient's Charter also set out certain expectations, which may or may not have been realistic. Prior to the implementation of the NHS Complaints Procedure on 1st April 1996, there had been a formal consultation by the Wilson Committee resulting in the publication 'Being Heard'.[4]

The guidance on implementation of the NHS Complaints Procedure was published in March 1996 and indicated that the legal frame work for this process would be based on a number of Directions to implement the new Complaints Procedure and that several regulations were being made that would affect the implementation including the National Health Service (General Medical Services) Amendment 1996.

There were a number of key objectives within the new procedure that included ease of access, simplification, and common features for complaints about services provided within the NHS. Importantly there was a separation of complaints from disciplinary procedures. The intention was to make it easier to extract lessons on quality from complaints in order to improve services provided and it is easy to see where the concept of clinical governance emanated from this principle. Also, the hope was that there would be fairness to staff and complainants alike with more rapid, open processes and a degree of honesty and thoroughness. The prime intention was not only to resolve the problem but also to satisfy the concerns raised by the complainant.

It was intended that there would be a move away from a confrontational, adversarial approach into a process that was much more of an investigative one and the overall concept was of the type found within alternative dispute resolution which has found great favour within the legal profession who are becoming increasingly aware of the disadvantages of too legalistic an approach.

REASONS WHY PEOPLE COMPLAIN

In general, a complaint results because an individual patient is dissatisfied with the management of their presenting condition by the doctor concerned. There are very few truly vexatious complaints and normally one can understand the reason why a patient is unhappy although, in fact, there may be no basis in reality for this and a simple explanation is quite capable of avoiding progression of the complaint.

Typically, there will have been an incident where there has been a communication problem or a degree of friction and with the benefit of hindsight it is often possible to establish why there has been a breakdown in the doctor–patient relationship resulting in them feeling the need to express their concern about what has happened to them. The doctor involved has the advantage of medical knowledge and even with the advent of Internet and various self-help telephone lines, it is quite possible to confuse the average patient unintentionally (e.g. by referring to a cerebrovascular accident rather than a stroke). Also, as part of their disease process the patient may not be able to appreciate an explanation given, particularly when the time set aside for the consultation has been truncated for whatever reason. Often, a thoughtful description of the illness in question with any possible side effects of treatment being put forward in a sensitive manner coupled with a willingness to answer queries is all that is required and it is rare indeed for a truly malicious complaint to be manufactured by a patient.

Complaints about doctors may arise through a number of routes:

- NHS hospital complaint
- NHS general practitioner(GP) complaint
- Ombudsman
- Civil litigation
- GMC
- Criminal prosecution
- Fatal Accident Inquiry/Coroner's Inquest.

Of course, not only may a doctor be required to submit to one of these processes but also an unlucky practitioner can end up going through all of these either simultaneously or sequentially.

Normally, MDOs will look after the professional interests of doctors and dentists whereas the British Medical Association (BMA) will assist with issues of personal conduct although it is quite possible that there is overlap. It is not unknown where a doctor is not, perhaps, a member of the BMA for their MDO to exercise their discretionary function by helping in this area.

Since the inception of the NHS Complaints Procedure, the number of disciplinary hearings has fallen dramatically, certainly, compared to the previous Terms of Service hearings where general practitioners were often involved in an acrimonious exchange with complainants who were present at the same time in a quasi legal setting. It is now unusual for more than 1% of NHS complaints to subsequently end up with the disciplinary hearing although this is still possible. Indeed, one of the principles of the new NHS Complaints Procedure was to separate entirely the complaints process from discipline.

However, as already indicated, there has been a marked growth in GMC complaints and whereas previously the GMC would write back to the complainant recommending that the NHS Complaints Procedure had not yet been exhausted, they are now often used as the first stop by a complainant. The GMC usually takes the matter forward if they feel there are concerns either about the doctor's conduct, i.e. that their failing constitutes serious professional misconduct, or that there is significant cause for concern by way of that doctor's performance.

Each year in England and Wales, there are a number of cases where the degree of recklessness is supposedly so gross that they result in a doctor being tried for manslaughter[5] and one such instance concerned an alleged loss of control in the insertion of a Hickman line in a patient with leukaemia where there was an undetected perforation of the atrium.[5] Thus far in Scotland there has only been one comparable case where a doctor's management of a patient with severe trigeminal neuralgia by way of a diamorphine injection ended with a High Court case for culpable homicide.[6]

Clearly, one of the attractive elements of pursuing a serious case through the criminal justice system for a patient is a direct accountability and specific punishment of perceived wrongdoing by the doctor. There is no doubt though that due to the enormous cost on the public purse, considerable consideration is given by the Crown Prosecution Service by way of instructing (hopefully) relevant expert opinion and also, perhaps, taking a view from leading counsel on the likelihood of a conviction as to whether it is, indeed, in the public interest to go ahead in the particular case in question.

Of course, in the civil courts the burden of proof is on the balance of probabilities i.e. whether or not one can reach 51% whereas in the criminal courts this is more difficult to quantify in that the case has to be proved by the prosecution 'beyond reasonable doubt'. Also, a case of this seriousness in the criminal sphere has to be considered by a jury whereas in the civil courts it would very much be the exception rather than the rule.

Should a doctor be found guilty of a criminal offence within the UK there is an automatic referral to the GMC and here the findings of the court are taken as proved and the case will not be re-heard by the Professional Conduct Committee (PCC). However they will allow representation made on behalf of the medical practitioner and reach a decision as to whether any additional sanction should be taken against the individual concerned.

FRAMEWORK OF THE COMPLAINT

A number of directions have been made to implement the 'new' Complaints Procedure along with a variety of regulations that affect the way in which this will be effected.

The view was taken that use of the patient's personal information to investigate a complaint was something where it was unnecessary to obtain the patient's express consent although care should be taken by the doctor to avoid disclosure of any incidental information and also to ensure that there is compliance with the GMC guidance contained within their booklet Confidentiality: Protecting and Providing Information.[7]

Obviously, where a complaint is made on behalf of a patient who has not specifically authorised another individual to act for him/her, caution should be exercised not to disclose personal health information to the complainant but the advice given by MDOs is that one should not be deemed obstructive although it may be valid to 'flag up' this particular issue.

Third parties who are not health care professionals who are identifiable from the patient's records should be protected in order to ensure compliance with the Data Protection Act 1998, although the guidance suggests that the consent of that individual can be overridden if the public interest justifies this. Where anonymous information will suffice then identifiable information should be omitted.

When the initial guidance came out, the relevant statute in respect to the mechanism of disclosure of clinical notes was the Access to Health Records Act 1990 although this has now been superseded in relation to living people by the Data Protection 1998. It was made clear that a complainant may use the NHS procedure to make a complaint about a subject access request rather than having to go to court, which would be a rather more cumbersome alternative. This continues to be the case although the Act of Parliament now specifies the right to approach the court to have inaccurate data rectified, blocked, erased, or destroyed.

Consideration was given to mixed sector complaints e.g. with Social Services Complaints Procedure, Mental Health Act Commissions Complaints Jurisdiction/Mental Welfare Commission. Although NHS bodies and local authorities were advised to ensure that all matters of concern to the complainant are in practise responded to under one or other procedure, the tendency in recent years has been to have multi-disciplinary enquiries internally or an independent external review which may not necessarily have the required safeguards for the practitioners concerned.

In regard to coroner's cases or Fatal Accident Inquiries, the fact that a death is under consideration by these agencies does not mean that all investigations into a complaint need to be suspended but the usual practise is to await their deliberations in order not to prejudice such a process.

There is increasing use made of private health care especially in England and Wales and although the complaints procedure will cover any complaint made about a Trust staff or facilities relating to that Trust's private pay beds, this does not extend to the private medical care provided by the consultant outwith his NHS contract. Since the inception of the NHS Complaints Procedure, there has been an increasing tendency for such cases simply to be referred to the GMC in the first instance.

THE COMPLAINTS PROCESS

This route of accountability is a formal procedure and an obligation was placed on the Trust/Health Board/Family Health Service Practitioners to establish the procedure and take steps to publicise the arrangements.

However, from 1 October 2002 responsibility for dealing with the independent review element of complaint about Family Health Service Practitioners passed from Health Authorities or Health Boards to Primary Care Trusts or Primary Care Groups depending on whether the doctor was based in Scotland or England and Wales.

Within the NHS there is a separate grievance procedure designed to address staff grievances and this continued to exist separately with clarification also being provided that disputes on contractual matters between Trusts and Practitioners would not be handled through the Complaints Procedure. Having said this, practitioners have the opportunity to complain to the Health Service Commissioner (Ombudsman) about the way in which they have been dealt with under the complaints procedure so this right of appeal applies to the respondent as much as the complainant.

One of the likely reasons for the marked increase in complaints experienced by medical defence organisations was the necessity for Trusts to ensure that the right to complain is well publicised to all patients, visitors, and staff. Consequently, it is now the norm in visiting an optician, general practitioner, or hospital outpatients to see reference to the process.

Complainants will exist or former patients and complaints may be made on behalf of them by anyone who has that person's consent. Curiously, if the patient is unable to act, then consent is not required. Should the Complaints Manager, or the Convenor at the Independent Review Panel stage not accept that the complainant is a suitable representative of a patient who is unable to give consent then they may refuse to deal with that individual and nominate another person to act on the patient's behalf. Certainly, these last two categories are exceptional and bearing in mind the ethos of the procedure is to try and reach a speedy resolution where that is possible, encouragement is given to try and achieve this.

There is a time limit on initiating complaints and a complaint should normally be made within six months of the incident resulting in the dissatisfaction, or within six months of the date of becoming aware of that problem, provided that is within 12 months of the problem. However, there is discretion that, more often than not, can be invoked to extend this time limit. At first glance this may appear unfair on the doctor but one has to realise that although there are proposals to restrict the GMC's ability to look into complaints outwith the previous five years except in exceptional circumstances, the NHS Complaints Procedure is considerably less stressful than the GMC and it may be in the respondent's best interests to submit to this route of accountability even if technically it would be possible to dispute that.

There is a requirement on the Trust to have a designated Complaints Manager who is readily accessible to the public and complainants must be able to refer complaints to them. Their primary role is to oversee the complaints procedure although the detailed role and functions should be decided by the Trust.

Family Health Service practices must have one person to administer the Complaints Procedure and that individual should be identifiable to patients and clients. Initially, this was often a partner in the practise but the tendency now is much more often to have the Practice Manager fulfil this function and their administrative background is of considerable value in ensuring the appropriate documentation is produced and that timescales are met.

If a personal response is in order then a simple explanation may often resolve that patient's concern but there is a recognised route of appeal should the preliminary response not address the complaint to the complainant's satisfaction. To that end, Trusts are required to appoint at least one person to act in the role of the Convenor to whom such requests are made.

One of the points emphasised in the new process was to separate complaints from discipline in order that appropriate lessons might be learned without the threat of sanction. It was stipulated that the purpose of the Complaints Procedure was not to apportion blame amongst staff but rather to investigate complaints to the satisfaction of the complainants while being scrupulously fair to staff. Having said this, there was a recognition that inevitably some complaints will identify information about serious issues necessitating disciplinary investigation.

Doctors have subsequently been made aware in the GMC document Management in Health Care: The Role of Doctors published in December 1999 that the first consideration for all managers must be the interests and safety of patients. Doctors must take action if they believe that patients are at risk of serious harm by way of a colleagues conduct, performance, or health and it unequivocally states in this document that concerns about a patient may arise from critical incident reporting or complaints from patients and doctors who receive such information have a duty to act on it.

While it is clearly stated that the Complaints Procedure should cease if the complainant explicitly indicates an intention to take legal action in respect to the complaint there is no doubt that a number of complainants use the process as a 'dry run' in order to obtain the necessary detail to litigate against that doctor or Trust. Oddly, there is nothing to stop a solicitor being instructed by a complainant to act for them in taking the preliminary steps within the procedure.

CONCILIATION

Conciliation is considered to be a voluntary process i.e. there has to be agreement by both parties to participate in this when it may yet be possible to resolve the complaint at a local level.

There is a requirement for lay conciliators to be made available by Trusts in order to optimise the conditions to achieve resolution. The intention of this process is to allow both parties to address the salient issues in a non-confrontational manner so that an acceptable agreement may be reached but not to impose a solution upon the parties concerned.

Confidentiality is integral to the conciliation process in order that the conciliator might encourage the participants to explore the reasons for the complaint in an open way. It is unequivocally stated that neither the conciliator nor the participants should provide information from

the process to any other person although it is in order for the conciliator to inform the Trust when conciliation has ceased and whether or
not it has been possible to reach a resolution.

While there is some flexibility within the system it is not normal to
have a representative from an MDO present. Likewise, it would be inappropriate for a solicitor to accompany a complainant although it would be
usual for them to have another individual there for support.

THE INDEPENDENT REVIEW PANEL

Complainants who are dissatisfied with the preliminary response may
refer a request for an Independent Review Panel to the Convenor either
orally or in writing within a period of 28 calendar days from the completion of the local resolution process.

It is necessary for the Convenor to obtain a statement signed by the complainant setting out the remaining grievances and why they are dissatisfied
with the outcome of local resolution. Thereafter, in deciding whether to
convene a Panel the Convenor has to consider, in consultation with an
independent lay chair from the regional list, whether the Trust can take
any further action short of establishing a Panel to satisfy the complainant
and also if establishing a Panel would add any further value to the process.

Although at first there was a tendency to acquiesce in a request to
hold such a hearing, this has now decreased so that only 22% of requests
in 2000–2001 resulted in a Panel going ahead.[8]

Where a complaint appears to relate either in whole or in part to clinical issues, the Convenor *must* take appropriate clinical advice in deciding whether to convene such a Panel.

The Convenor has to inform the complainant in writing of the decision taken as to whether or not a Panel should be appointed, setting out
clearly the terms of reference if a Panel has to be set up or the reasons
for any decision resulting in refusal. Should a complaint progress to this
stage then one of the things that a MDO requires from the doctor concerned is the terms of service as if there is significant divergence from
these it is possible to object.

Although it may appear biased in print, there is an obligation on the
Convenor to make the complainant aware of their right of appeal to the
Ombudsman if a Panel has been refused and there is no alternative in
this respect.

Independent Review Panels (IRPs) are composed of three lay members
and their function is to investigate the aspects of the complaint set out
in the terms of reference. The Panel has no executive authority over any
action by the Trust or Board. Further, it may not make any suggestion in

its report that any person should be subject to disciplinary action or referred to their professional regulatory bodies.

It is up to the Panel to decide how to conduct its proceedings having regard to guidance issued by the NHS within the following rules:

- The Panel's proceedings be held in private.
- The Panel must give both parties a reasonable opportunity to express their views.
- Should any of the Panel members disagree how the Panel should go about its business, the Chairman's decision will be final.

When being interviewed by the Panel the complainant and any other person interviewed may be accompanied by a person of their choosing who, provided the Chairman agrees, may speak to the Panel except that no one may be accompanied by a legally qualified person acting as an advocate.

While there is some variation in approach as to how this functions in practice, there is normally not an impediment to a medico-legal adviser with a law degree actually assisting a doctor provided they are not a solicitor or advocate/barrister.

When the complaint is either wholly or partially related to clinical matters it is necessary for the Panel to be advised by *at least* two Independent Clinical Assessors and these will normally come from the specialty in question.

Following receipt of the Panel's report, the Chief Executive of the Trust must write to the complainant informing them of any action they propose to take as a result of the Panel's deliberations and of the right of the complainant to take their grievance to the Ombudsman if they remain dissatisfied.

The intention is that the report should have a restricted circulation to those involved but, of course, it is not unknown for the complainant to then pass this to the media and a report to appear in the public domain thereafter.

There are various time limits set out within the guidance and it is safe to say there is often difficulty in achieving these targets (only 9% of IRPs were concluded within target in 2000–2001) although with greater familiarity progress is being made to reach them.

THE OMBUDSMAN

Whereas previously the Health Service Commissioner was predominately involved in looking at cases of mal-administration often in respect to the handling of a complaint, from 31st March 1996 the Ombudsman was also able to investigate complaints about clinical issues both in hospital or general practice.

SUMMARY

A variety of routes of accountability have been set out but the one that a doctor practising within the UK is most likely to face is the NHS Complaints Procedure and subsequent to April 1996 this has almost certainly achieved the purpose of providing a thorough investigation of the issues raised albeit not always to the entire satisfaction of the complainant.

The previous confrontational and legalistic process has by and large been dispensed with and although there are still inherent delays in the system, particularly in the hospital sector, the complainant is usually able to obtain a better understanding of the medical management of their care that is within the ethos of clinical governance allowing doctors to learn from adverse events in order that their practise might subsequently be improved.

Of course, there continues to be safeguards for society generally where that doctor's conduct may be so serious that GMC intervention is justified or their performance is so seriously deficient that it is necessary for this to be examined.

If doctors are to be allowed to continue to self-regulate, this being one of the hallmarks of a profession, there is a requirement to be accountable. However, the hope is that if the NHS Complaints Procedure can be refined this may avoid complainants deciding to have a number of further bites at the cherry through the other routes open to them.

REFERENCES AND FURTHER READING

1. *Hunter v Hanley*, 1955, SC 200, 1955 SLT 213.
2. *Bolam v Friern HMC*, 1957, 2 All ER 118; 1957, 1 WLR 582, 101 Sol Jo 357, 1 BMLR 1.
3. Personal Communication. The Medical and Dental Defence Union of Scotland, 1997.
4. The Report of a Review Committee on NHS Complaints Procedures, 1994, *Being Heard*, Department of Health.
5. *R v Woodburn*, 2001, *The Times*, 22 December.
6. *HM Advocate v Watson*, 1991, Scotsman, 11 June, p. 8, 14 June, p. 3.
7. *Confidentiality: Protecting and Providing Information*, The General Medical Council, 2000.
8. National Statistics, *Handling Complaints: Monitoring the NHS Complaints Procedures*. England, Financial Year 2000–2001.

8

The Mental Health Act (England and Wales)

Alain Gregoire

The Mental Health Act 1983 relates to issues of consent to treatment and admission of mentally disordered people in England and Wales. This Act of Parliament is divided into 10 parts (Box 8.1) and 149 sections. Only a few of these are immediately relevant to common clinical practise and these will be considered in this chapter. For the purposes of the Act, mental disorder is divided into three broad categories:

1 Mental illness: not specifically defined by promiscuity
2 Mental impairment or severe mental impairment: defined in terms of impairment of intelligence and social function when associated with abnormally aggressive or seriously irresponsible conduct
3 Psychopathic disorder: persistent disorder or disability of mind which results in abnormally aggressive or seriously irresponsible conduct (with or without impairment of intelligence).

THE MENTAL HEALTH ACT COMMISSION

The Mental Health Act Commission is a statutory body appointed by the Secretary of State to oversee and regulate the correct application of

---

Box 8.1 The 10 parts of the Mental Health Act 1983.

Part I: Defines mental disorder
Part II: Civil Detention Orders and Guardianship
Part III: Criminal Justice Orders
Part IV: Consent to treatment
Part V: Mental Health Tribunals
Part VI: Movement of patients in and out of England and Wales
Part VII: Court of Protection
Part VIII: Duties of local authorities and the Secretary of State
Part IX: Offences
Part X: Miscellaneous provisions.

Box 8.2 Glossary.

ASW: Approved Social Worker – qualified to make applications for
   detention under the Act
MHAC: Mental Health Act Commission
MHRT: Mental Health Review Tribunal
RMO: Responsible Medical Officer – Doctor (consultant) in charge of
   patient's care
Section 12(2) Approved Doctor: Doctor with experience of psychiatry
   and approved by the Region to make medical recommendations under
   the Act
SOAD: Second Opinion Approved Doctor – psychiatrist appointed by
   MHAC.

---

the Act. The Commission consists of a panel of psychiatrists, nurses, social workers, lawyers and members of the lay public under the chairmanship of a lawyer. Their duties include preparing a Code of Practice,[1] visiting all psychiatric hospitals and registered mental homes, scrutinising documents relating to the detention of patients under the Act and investigating complaints. They appoint Second Opinion Approved Doctors (SOADs – see Box 8.2). They are now also involved in overseeing the proper application of supervision registers and the care programme approach.

Civil detention order

These include the longer term treatment orders (Sections 3 and 7) and the briefer orders for assessment (Sections 2, 4, 5, 135, 136).

Section 2: Admission for assessment

This allows compulsory admission for up to 28 days, for assessment or assessment followed by treatment for mental disorder. This order is appropriate when the patient is not well known to the service or when the diagnosis or most appropriate management are not established. The formalities involve application by the patient's nearest relative or preferably an Approved Social Worker (ASW), supported by two medical recommendations. The latter *must* include at least one Section 12 approved doctor and one doctor with previous acquaintance of the patient (usually the patient's general practitioner); if this is not possible it is desirable for both doctors to be Section 12 approved. The following grounds must apply:

1 The patient is suffering from a mental disorder of a nature or degree which warrants such detention *and* the admission is

necessary in the interests of the patient's own health *or* safety or for the protection of others.

2 The ASW and doctors should also satisfy themselves that alternative forms of care or treatment, including informal admission are not possible. They have a professional responsibility to ensure that they obtain as much information as possible about the patient and that they discuss the patient with each other. It is the doctors' responsibility to ensure that a hospital bed will be available. Admission to hospital must take place within 14 days of the latest medical recommendation. No more than 5 days must elapse between the doctors' examination of the patient.

Section 2 cannot be reviewed. If continued detention is necessary Section 3 should be considered.

Section 4: Emergency admission for assessment

This allows compulsory admission for up to 72 hours for assessment and should only be used in emergency situations in the community when the delay in obtaining a second opinion for a Section 2 admission would result in a significant risk of harm to the patient or others, or serious harm to property. Only one medical recommendation from a registered medical practitioner is required. Application can be made by nearest relative or preferably by an ASW. The latter must satisfy themselves that the situation is a genuine emergency and that there are adequate grounds for proceeding without a second doctor. The convenience of any of those involved does not constitute adequate grounds. Both the applicant and the doctor must have seen the patient within the previous 24 hours and the doctor should preferably know the patient. Admission must take place within 24 hours of completion of the earliest form.

Unlike Sections 2 and 3, this Section does not allow for compulsory treatment (except under common law). A second medical opinion must be obtained as soon as possible with a view to converting to a Section 2. Social Services should be informed of this, although the original ASW remains valid. The Section 2 is then valid for 28 days from when the Section 4 took effect.

Section 5: Detection of informal inpatients

This allows for the emergency detention of an informal inpatient in a hospital or registered nursing home for the purposes of an assessment with a view to a Section 2 or 3. Section 5(4) is the nurse's holding power which may be used by a registered mental health nurse if a registered medical practitioner is not immediately available. This has a maximum duration of six hours and expires upon arrival of the Responsible Medical Officer's (RMO's) nominated deputy who should attend as soon as possible. Section 5(2) may be used by the RMO's deputy to detain an informal inpatient, or an inpatient held under Section 5(4) for the purposes of an assessment. This Section has a maximum duration of 72 hours. However, it should not be allowed to expire, as an assessment should have been carried out prior to that time. The Section 5(2) ceases to apply from the moment that assessment has been completed and the patient therefore becomes informal unless another section of the Act is applied.

Section 135

Section 135 is a magistrate's warrant allowing an ASW entry to a private residence to remove a person thought to be suffering from a mental disorder and who has been, or is being, ill-treated, neglected or kept otherwise than under proper control or is unable to care for himself and is living alone. The person is conveyed to a place of safety for up to 72 hours for the purpose of an assessment by registered medical practitioners and ASW.

Section 136: Mentally disordered persons found in public places

Section 136 allows a police officer to remove to a place of safety any person who appears to be suffering from a mental disorder in a place to which the public has access. The person must appear to be in immediate need of care and control and such action must appear necessary in the person's interest or for the protection of others. A maximum of 72 hours is allowed, during which the person must be assessed by an ASW *and* a registered medical practitioner. Local policy must be agreed between Social Services, Health Services and the police in all areas.

Section 3: Admission for treatment

Under Section 3, compulsory admission is allowed for up to 6 months for treatment. The same requirements for medical recommendations apply as for Section 2. Applications can be made by nearest relative or (preferably) by an ASW who must make every effort to contact the nearest relative. The ASW cannot proceed with the application if the nearest relative objects. However, a County Court can transfer the powers of the nearest relative if it considers the objection to be unreasonable. The following grounds must apply:

1 The patient is suffering from a mental illness, severe mental illness, psychopathic disorder or mental impairment; one of these categories must be specified and agreed by both doctors and applicant *and*
2 The mental disorder is of a degree which makes is appropriate for the patient to receive treatment in hospital *and*
3 It is necessary in the interests of his health or safety or for the protection of others that he receives such treatment and it cannot be provided unless he is detained, *and*
4 In the case of mental impairment or psychopathic disorder, such treatment is likely to alleviate or prevent a deterioration in his condition. The same time limits as for Section 2 apply to the completion of documents. Section 3 is renewable by the RMO for 6 months in the first instance, and then yearly if the grounds for admission continue to apply.

Section 7: Guardianship

Under Section 7 a guardian, normally had the local authority social services department, is empowered to require the patient to:

1 live at a specified place
2 attend for outpatient treatment, occupation, education or training (although there is no power to enforce cooperation or compliance with such interventions)
3 permit access to himself at the place where he is living.

Requirements for application are as for Section 3 and the patient must be 16 years of age or over. Duration and renewal is as for Section 3.

Unless the patient recognises the authority of the Guardian and as a result cooperates with the Guardian, this Order conveys little benefit. The Code of Practice states that if there is consistent lack of compliance the Order should be discharged. The Order is little used, and it is debatable whether it is under-used.

PATIENTS CONCERNED IN CRIMINAL PROCEEDINGS (PART III OF THE ACT)

Patients awaiting trial

Section 35 allows the remand of an accused person to hospital for a report for 28 days, renewable for up to 12 weeks. One medical recommendation from a Section 12 approved doctor is required, in addition to a court order. Crown Courts may apply this order to any person awaiting trial for an imprisonable offence. In Magistrates' Courts the person must be convicted or awaiting sentence, or the court must be satisfied that he committed the act or made the omission or he must consent to the exercise of the power.

Section 36: Remand to hospital for treatment

Section 36 permits a Crown Court accompanied by two medical recommendations (one of them by an approved doctor) to remand an accused person to hospital for treatment up to 28 days renewable for up to 12 weeks.

Convicted offenders

Section 37: Hospital Admission or Guardianship Order

This provides the court with an alternative to imprisonment or other punishment and has the same effect as applying a Section 3 or Guardianship Order. Once it is implemented the court has no further involvement with the patient. The Order requires that the same grounds as for Section 3 apply to the patient *and* that the court is satisfied that this is the most suitable method of disposing the case and that the court has two medical recommendations (one from an approved doctor) and, in the case of a hospital order, that the hospital has agreed to admit the patient.

Section 48

The Home Secretary also has the power to transfer such persons to hospital when urgent treatment is required. A Restriction Order (see below) is applied for people detained in prison on remand.

Section 38: Interim Hospital Order

Under Section 38 two medical recommendations are required (one from an approved doctor *and* one from the admitting hospital) that the person is suffering from mental illness, psychopathic disorder, severe mental impairment or mental impairment such that the hospital order may be appropriate *and* that he will be admitted within 28 days. This can be converted to a Section 37 by the court at any stage.

Section 47: Home Secretary's power to transfer sentenced prisoners

Section 47 allows the Home Secretary, on the basis of two written medical recommendations (one from an approved doctor) to transfer a convicted offender to hospital. The doctors must agree on the form of mental disorder as for Section 3. The Home Secretary can order the person back to prison at any time.

Restricted Detention Orders

Section 41: Order restricting discharge

Such an order is applied in addition to Section 37 (Section 37/41) by a Crown Court after considering:

- the nature of the offence
- antecedents of the offender
- risk of further offences
- protection of the public.

The court must have heard oral evidence from at least one of the medical practitioners. The Restriction Order has the effect of giving the Home Secretary the responsibility for granting leave and allowing discharge with or without limit of time. The RMO must request permission from the Home Secretary for any leave (except within hospital grounds), transfer or discharge. The Hospital Order (Section 37) does not expire or require renewal while the Section 41 is in force. Patients can be conditionally discharged, the Section 41 remaining in place, and must abide by conditions imposed by the Home Office. Breaking conditions can lead to readmission under Section 37/41. Informal admission of Section 41 patients is also possible.

Section 49: Restriction of prisoners transferred to hospital

Section 49 has the same effect as Section 41 but is applied to Section 47 (Section 47/49). This can be terminated at any time by the Home Secretary and expires when the fixed term of the prisoner's sentence ends. Applications can be made to the Home Secretary for discharge.

PART IV OF THE ACT: CONSENT TO TREATMENT

Part IV applies to patients detained under all sections of the Act *except* Sections 4, 5(4), 5(2), 135, 136, patients in a place of safety under

Section 37 pending admission to hospital, and patients subject to Section 7 (guardianship). The provisions allow for the administration of reversible medical treatments (medication or Electro-Convulsive Therapy, ECT) without consent for up to 3 months to patients detained under a section to which this part applies. However, consent must first be sought in all patients. The provisions apply only to medical treatment for mental disorder. Treatment of physical disorder can only lawfully be given under the Act if this is necessary to alleviate the mental disorder.

Section 57: Treatments requiring the patient's consent and a second opinion (from a SOAD)

This applies at present only to psychosurgery and surgical hormone implantation to reduce male sex-drive. This safeguard applies also to informal patients.

Section 58: Treatments requiring consent or a second opinion

Section 58 applies to patients who have been treated with medication for 3 months (with or without consent) and to any detained patient requiring ECT. Consent must be certified by the RMO or Section 12 approved doctor, or a SOAD must agree to the treatment plan.

Section 62

In urgent situations, when immediately necessary, reversible treatments may be given without consent under the direction of the RMO.

Section 63

A range of therapeutic interventions are covered by Section 63, such as nursing care, occupational therapy or behaviour therapy for which consent should be sought but is not required. However, such interventions are unlikely to be particularly effective without some degree of cooperation.

PART V: RIGHTS OF APPEAL

Hospital managers have a duty to inform patients of their rights verbally and in writing at the beginning of a compulsory admission. These include information about the detention order, consent to treatment, rights of appeal and complaints procedures. Rights of appeal and nearest relative's rights are summarised in Table 8.1. Patients detained under Sections 2, 3 or 37 may appeal to the managers as often as they wish.

Table 8.1 Rights of appeal to Mental Health Review Tribunals.		
Section	*Rights of appeal*	
	By patient	*By nearest relative*
Section 2	within 14 days	none
Section 3*	to MHRT – in first 6 months	none
Guardianship	to MHRT – in first 6 months	none
Section 37**	after 6 months, then yearly	after 6 months, then yearly
Section 37/41	after 6 months, then yearly	none

* Automatic appeal after 6 months without an MHRT hearing, and 3-yearly thereafter.
** Automatic appeal after 3 years' detention without an MHRT hearing.
Patients detained under Sections 2, 3 and 37 may appeal to Hospital Managers as often as they wish.

The Mental Health (Patients in the Community) Act 1995

Mental health services in the UK have undergone a considerable shift of emphasis from inpatient care to care outside hospitals. However, the Mental Health Act 1983 is almost entirely hospital-focused and it has become increasingly apparent that the Act fails to meet the needs of patients and professionals in the community setting.[5,6,7] Enforced treatment of patients in the community has been opposed as an infringement of human rights,[8] but it is arguable that the current situation, which involves enforced treatment combined with hospitalisation, is a greater infringement, particularly in the case of patients who only require the treatment and not necessarily the hospitalisation. A tentative legislative move in this direction occurred with the Mental Health (Patients in the Community) Act 1995 which gives key workers (normally Community Psychiatric Nurses, CPNs) powers in the community, including the power to require patients to live in a specified place and attend for treatment, and to seek the RMO's review with a view to recall to hospital if they fail to comply with medication (Section 25).

Such measures have been criticised as introducing or even imposing coercive practices on professionals without giving them adequate power simply to treat patients[9] and the use of this legislation has varied greatly between services.

The Human Rights Act 1998

The Human Rights Act 1998 incorporates most of the articles of the European Convention on Human Rights and came into force in October 2000. The articles of particular relevance to mental health law are listed in Box 8.3.

Box 8.3 Most relevant articles of the Human Rights Act to mental health.

- Article 2: Right to life
- Article 3: Prohibition of torture or inhuman or degrading treatment or punishment
- Article 5: Right to liberty and security of person (exceptions include lawful detention of persons of unsound mind but stipulates entitlement to appeal proceedings to be decided speedily by a Court)
- Article 6: Right to a fair trial within a reasonable period of time by an independent and impartial tribunal established by law
- Article 8: Right to respect for private and family life, home and correspondence.

As a result of the Act, the procedures involved in implementing various parts of the Mental Health Act have been challenged in a number of cases, some successfully. These relate to such areas as delays to hearing of appeals (Article 5), inhuman treatment (Article 3) and homicide by a mentally ill person (Article 2). A range of potential challenges by mentally ill people to the care they receive are likely, although European cases so far suggest that good clinical practise in this area is usually compatible with the requirements of the Human Rights Act.[10]

Proposed new legislation

The Government has published its proposals for a new mental health law to replace the 1983 Mental Health Act in a White Paper issued in 2000 followed by a draft Bill published in 2002.[11] The proposed legislation has been met with almost universal criticism from involved parties such as the Royal College of Psychiatrists, the Law Society, patient and carer groups and voluntary organisations. These groups formed a unique alliance to raise their serious concerns about the overall emphasis on public protection and numerous specific elements of the proposed legislation (Box 8.4).

Promised publication of responses to the draft Bill by the Government has so far not occurred and it is not clear as yet to the parties involved what the Government response to the consultation is likely to be. Meanwhile, in Scotland, a new Mental Health Bill has been passed which, both in process and final outcome, has generally met with the approval of most parties involved.

Box 8.4 Principle criticisms of Draft Mental Health Bill for England and Wales.

- Reduces existing restrictions on detention
  - Diagnosis need not be specified (single term 'mental disorder')
  - No specific exclusion criteria (such as substance misuse, sexual behaviour or neurological disorders)
  - Severity ('degree') only needs to be sufficient to warrant medical treatment (not necessarily specialist or inpatient)
  - Patient does not have to be considered treatable (but appropriate treatment must be available)
- Treatment orders (i.e. over 28 days) will automatically need ratification by tribunals in all cases
- Tribunals can impose restrictions on RMO's ability to allow leave or discharge patients (this, therefore, may lead to compulsion of professionals and services to provide care which neither patients nor professionals believe is necessary).
- Duty on National Health Service Trusts to provide assessment under the Act of any person at the request of any person
- The additional resources, in particular Consultant Psychiatrists of which there is a national shortage, will be diverted from clinical care to implement this legislation.
- The implicit and explicit emphasis on the protection of the public from mentally ill people will damage the efforts that are being made by all parties, including Government agencies, to reduce the stigma associated with mental illness and mental health services.

CONCLUSIONS

The Mental Health Act 1983 provides the legal framework for the difficult balancing act between the basic human and civil rights of mentally ill individuals on the one hand, and on the other their right to receive treatment for severe mental illness and the need to protect them and other members of society from the effects of such illness.[2,3,4] The use of the Mental Health Act should never replace attempts to gain patients' cooperation with treatment through the development of good relations, discussion, education, persuasion, compromise and bargaining. Failure to explore adequate alternative forms of management goes against the spirit of the Act.

Community care offers considerable benefits to the majority of individuals with mental illness through flexible, needs-led approaches to management combined with effective systems for assessing those needs and delivering and monitoring care. However, an important minority of patients with chronic symptoms remain disturbed, vulnerable and occasionally dangerous, and require very considerable resources which may not always be available. Thus we continue to see the appalling personal and social consequences of severe mental illness, and the resulting media coverage leads to dramatic criticisms of community care and demands for greater legislative powers to control the mentally ill. It is to be hoped that the Government will introduce new legislation that improves the quality and safety of care through measures which satisfy the aspirations and concerns of the major stakeholders involved.

REFERENCES

1. Department of Health and Welsh office. *Code of Practice, Mental Health Act 1983*. London: HMSO, 1993.
2. Department of Health and Social Security. *Mental Health Act 1983*, Memorandum on Parts I–IV, VIII and X. London: HMSO, 1983.
3. Gostin L. *A Practical Guide to Mental Health Law*. London: MIND, 1983.
4. Royal Commission on the laws relating to mental illness and mental deficiencies. Report. London: HMSO, 1957.
5. Turner T. Community care. *Brit. J. Psychiat.*, 1988, 152: 1–3.
6. Royal College of Psychiatrists. *Community Treatment Orders: A Discussion Document*. London: Royal College of Psychiatrists, 1993.
7. Royal College of Psychiatrists. *Community Supervision Orders*. London: Royal College of Psychiatrists, 1993.
8. House of Commons Health Committee. *Community Supervision Orders*. Health Committee 5th report, volume 1. London: HMSO, 1993.
9. Eastman N. Anti-therapeutic community mental health law. *Brit. Med. J.*, 1995, 310: 1081–1082.
10. MacGregor-Morris R, Ewbank J, Birmingham L. Potential impact of the Human Rights Act on psychiatric practice: the best of British values? *Brit. Med. J.*, 2001, 322: 848–850.
11. Department of Health. *Draft Mental Health Bill*. London: Stationery Office, 2002.

9

Death certification and the role of the coroner

Peter Dean

CORONERS – PAST, PRESENT AND FUTURE

Since the first edition of this book, a number of very significant events, such as the trial and subsequent conviction of Dr Harold Shipman and separate concerns about organ retention following enquiries into events at Alder Hey and other hospitals, have focused the attention of the legal and medical professions and the general public itself on the processes involved in the investigation of sudden death.

The nature of the coronership at present is that it responds to and investigates those deaths which have been referred to it for a wide variety of reasons (just over one third of all deaths in England and Wales at the present time), rather than pro-actively screening all deaths that occur, whether in the community or in hospital, and then determining which ones should be subjected to further scrutiny.

The latter approach is not allowed by the law as it currently stands but, in the wake of Dr Shipman's conviction, there have been three separate enquiries examining the way in which sudden death is investigated, and it is likely that there will ultimately be new legislation and subsequent changes to the way in which all deaths are investigated and the manner in which coroners carry out their duties. Some of the proposals which have been made will be touched on at the end of this chapter but, initially this chapter will review how the office of coroner developed, the current law and practice, and some of the changes that have occurred in recent years.

HISTORICAL DEVELOPMENT

It is in the general interests of the community that any sudden, unnatural or unexplained deaths should be investigated, and to reflect this, the role of the coroner has adapted over the eight centuries since the office was formally established in 1194, from being a form of medieval tax gatherer to an independent judicial officer charged with the investigation of sudden, violent or unnatural death.[1]

The duties of the early coroners were varied, and included the investigation of almost any aspect of medieval life that had the potential benefit of revenue for the Crown. Suicides were investigated, on the grounds that the goods and chattels of those found guilty of the crime of 'felo de se' or 'self murder' would then be forfeit to the Crown, as were wrecks of the sea, fires, both fatal and non-fatal, and any discovery of buried treasure in the community, which is still on the statute books today as 'treasure trove'. Sudden death in the community had always been considered important and was also investigated, although for reasons far different to those of today.

After the Norman Conquest, to deter the local communities from a continuing habit of killing Normans, a heavy fine was levied on any village where a dead body was discovered, on the assumption that it was presumed to be Norman, unless it could be proved to be English. The fine was known as the 'Murdrum', from which the word 'murder' is derived and, as the system developed, many of the early coroners' inquests dealt with the 'Presumption of Normanry' which could only be rebutted by the local community, and a fine thus avoided, by the 'Presentment of Englishry'.

The coroner system continued to adapt over the centuries, but in the nineteenth century major changes relating to the investigation of death in the community occurred. In 1836, the first Births and Deaths Registration Act was passed, prompted by the public concern and panic caused by inaccurate 'parochial' recording of the actual numbers of deaths arising from epidemics such as cholera.

There was also growing concern that given the easy and uncontrolled access to numerous poisons, and inadequate medical investigation of the actual cause of death, many homicides were going undetected.

By then, the coroner's fiscal responsibility had diminished and the Coroners Act of 1887 made significant changes here, repealing much of the earlier legislation. Coroners then became more concerned with determining the circumstances and the actual medical causes of sudden, violent, and unnatural deaths for the benefit of the community as a whole.

DEATH CERTIFICATION

Section 22 of the Births and Deaths Registration Act 1953[2] provides that

> In the case of the death of any person who has been attended during his
> last illness by a registered medical practitioner, that practitioner shall sign

a certificate in the prescribed form stating to the best of his knowledge and belief the cause of death and shall forthwith deliver that certificate to the registrar.

Much unnecessary distress to grieving relatives waiting in a Register Office trying to register a death, and a great deal of subsequent anger directed at the individual doctor by those bereaved, can easily be avoided by taking care to ensure that the Medical Certificate of Cause of Death is completed properly and will not be rejected by the Registrar of Births and Deaths.

In the first instance this involves a knowledge and recognition of those deaths that must be reported to the coroner, as outlined below, in which case the coroner's office should be contacted by telephone for further guidance at the earliest possible opportunity prior to writing any certificate.

The Registrar of Births and Deaths scrutinises all Medical Certificates of Cause of Death, and has a statutory duty under Section 41(1) of the Registration of Births and Deaths Regulations 1987 to report the death to the coroner if it is one

- (a) in respect of which the deceased was not attended during his last illness by a registered medical practitioner; or
- (b) in respect of which the registrar
  - (i) has been unable to obtain a duly completed certificate of the cause of death; or
  - (ii) has received such a certificate with respect to which it appears to him, from the particulars contained in the certificate or otherwise, that the deceased was not seen by the certifying medical practitioner either after death or within 14 days before death; or
- (c) the cause of which appears to be unknown; or
- (d) which the registrar has reason to believe to have been unnatural or to have been caused by violence or neglect or by abortion, or to have been attended by suspicious circumstances; or
- (e) which appears to the registrar to have occurred during an operation or before recovery from the effect of an anaesthetic; or
- (f) which appears to the registrar from the contents of any medical certificate of cause of death to have been due to industrial disease or industrial poisoning.

Local arrangements usually exist for notifying deaths that occur within 24 hours of admission to hospital. This is not a statutory requirement, but the registrar may otherwise question a certificate if it appears that the patient may not have been in hospital long enough to enable the cause of death to be fully established, or if it appears that the patient was not attended during the last illness by a registered medical practitioner other than treatment given in extremis by hospital staff.

Section 41(1) of the Registration of Births and Deaths Regulations defines most of the instances when a death must be reported to the coroner. It does not cover absolutely every case, however, an exception being deaths in custody which, rather than being notified through the registrar, will be reported directly to the coroner by the appropriate prison or police authority. The medical practitioner must be aware, though, that a prisoner who dies while as a patient in hospital is still deemed legally to be in custody whether under guard or not, and such deaths must still be reported to the coroner, whether natural or not, rather than being registered in the normal manner.

Where the death is entirely natural and does not fall into any of the above categories, then to ensure that the Medical Certificate of Cause of Death is acceptable to the Registrar of Births and Deaths, care must be taken to ensure that the certificate is completed correctly, and the correct format employed. Useful advice on this was given in a letter to doctors from the Office of Population Censuses and Surveys in 1990.[3]

This reminded doctors that the certificates served both legal and statistical purposes, and pointed out some of the common errors in certification that occur. It specifically mentions that there is no need to record the mode of dying, as this does not assist in deriving mortality statistics, and stresses that it is even more important not to complete a certificate where the mode of dying, for example shock, uraemia or asphyxia, is the only entry.

It emphasises the need to avoid the use of abbreviations at all times. This can clearly be a source of ambiguity and confusion, particularly where abbreviations are shared, such as 'M.I.' which might mean mitral incompetence or myocardial infarction, or 'M.S.' which might mean mitral stenosis or multiple sclerosis.

Where the fatal disease process is one that is often recognised to be employment-related but is known not to be in that particular patient, then the addition of the words 'non-industrial' on the certificate after the cause of death can avoid subsequent enquiry by the registrar.

It is also worth noting that there are very useful notes and directions accompanying books of blank Medical Certificates of Cause of Death.[4] Following these will avoid many of the common problems that arise, for example relating to the correct inclusion and positioning of any relevant antecedent diseases or conditions, and will ensure that part I, and where appropriate part II, are filled in correctly and in a logical sequence.

Problems leading to the rejection of certificates frequently arise when junior doctors, uncertain of the exact cause of death or what they should write, are asked to complete the Medical Certificate of Cause of Death. If in any doubt they should always consult their senior colleagues in these circumstances. A survey however, revealed similar and significant numbers of failures to recognise which deaths are reportable across all grades of doctor from junior to senior.[5]

Any doctor who is uncertain therefore, regardless of seniority, would be best advised to seek the guidance of the local coroner's office to resolve any doubts and to avoid any subsequent problems and distress to relatives.

Aspects of transplantation are also discussed elsewhere in this book, but it is worthy of note that, in addition to the normal requirements relating to consent that must be satisfied prior to any transplant, by Section 1(5) of the Human Tissue Act 1961, the consent of the coroner must also be obtained prior to any transplant 'where a person has reason to believe that an inquest may be required to be held on any body or that a postmortem examination of any body may be required by the coroner'.

At the present time, as stated previously, just over a third of all deaths in England and Wales are reported to coroners. In 2002, out of a total of approximately 535,400 deaths, 201,389 were reported, and the outcome of these deaths will now be examined.

NATURAL DEATHS

In those circumstances where further enquiry indicates that a reported death is due to natural causes and does not require a postmortem examination, the coroner will issue a Form 100A, which notifies the registrar that the death was due to natural causes, and the attending doctor will be advised to complete a Medical Certificate of the Cause of Death in the usual manner.

In the majority of cases reported to coroners, however, a postmortem examination is still required to ascertain the cause of death, although the proportion of cases requiring this has been declining slowly over the years. If the cause of death is found to be natural at autopsy, the coroner will issue a Form 100B, which notifies the registrar of the cause of death, and that no further action is to be taken.

Upon receipt of either the Medical Certificate of the Cause of Death from the attending doctor, or Form 100B from the coroner, the registrar is able to register the death and issue a disposal certificate to allow for arrangements to be made to dispose of the body.

In 2002, postmortem examinations were conducted on 117,700 of the cases reported to coroners, representing just over 58 per cent of the

201,389 reported deaths and continuing a steady downward trend here. There has, however, been a steady increase in the number of cases where neither a postmortem examination nor an inquest has been required.

UNNATURAL DEATHS AND INQUESTS

In cases where the cause of death is found not to be natural, the coroner has a statutory duty to conduct an inquest under Section 8(1) of the Coroners Act 1988, which provides that:

> Where a coroner is informed that a body of a person ("the deceased") is lying within his district and there is reasonable cause to suspect that the deceased
>
> (a) has died a violent or unnatural death;
> (b) has died a sudden death of which the cause is unknown; or
> (c) has died in prison, or in such a place or in such circumstances as to require an inquest under any other Act,
>
> then, whether the cause of death arose within his district or not, the coroner shall as soon as practicable hold an inquest into the death of the deceased either with or, subject to subsection (3), without a jury.

The issue of what constituted an 'unnatural death' for the purposes of an inquest was explored by the Court of Appeal in R (Touche) v Inner North London Coroner, 2001 Q.B. 1206, CA.[6] Here a woman had died from severe hypertension and cerebral haemorrhage following the delivery of twins by Caesarean section, and there was medical evidence that the death would probably have been avoided had her blood pressure been monitored post-operatively. The Court of Appeal ruled that, even if a death was from what was essentially a recognised natural cause, it should be considered as potentially 'unnatural' for the purposes of an inquest if there was evidence that neglect could have contributed to the death.

Other cases in recent years have demonstrated the impact of the Human Rights Act 1998, particularly Article 2 dealing with the right to life, and have emphasized the importance of a thorough inquest in the investigation of deaths such as those in prison or police custody. Practice here is evolving as the case law in this area develops.

JURIES

Prior to 1926, every inquest had to be held with a jury, but nowadays, in the majority of inquests, the coroner sits alone. Section 8(3) of the

Coroners Act 1988 provides that:

> If it appears to a coroner, either before he proceeds to hold an inquest or in
> the course of an inquest begun without a jury, that there is reason to suspect
>
> (a) that the death occurred in prison or in such a place or in such
>   circumstances as to require an inquest under any other Act;
> (b) that the death occurred while the deceased was in police custody, or
>   resulted from an injury caused by a police officer in the purported
>   execution of his duty;
> (c) that the death was caused by an accident, poisoning or disease, notice
>   of which is required to be given under any Act to a government
>   department, to any inspector or other officer of a government
>   department or to an inspector appointed under Section 19 of the
>   Health and Safety at Work etc. Act 1974; or
> (d) that the death occurred in circumstances the continuance or
>   possible recurrence of which is prejudicial to the health or safety of
>   the public or any section of the public, he shall proceed to summon
>   a jury in the manner required by subsection (2).

PROCEDURES AT AN INQUEST

The conduct of an inquest is governed by The Coroners Rules 1984, and
the function and ambit of an inquest was usefully examined and clearly
re-affirmed by the Court of Appeal in R v North Humberside Coroner,
ex parte Jamieson, 1994, 3 W.L.R. 82.[7]

Rule 36 (Matters to be Ascertained at Inquest) provides that:

> (1) The proceedings and evidence at inquest shall be directed solely to
>   ascertaining the following matters, namely,
>   (a) who the deceased was;
>   (b) how, when and where the deceased came by his death;
>   (c) the particulars for the time being required by the Registration
>   Acts to be registered concerning the death
> (2) Neither the coroner nor the jury shall express any opinion on any
>   other matters.

and Rule 42 (Verdict) provides that:

> No verdict shall be framed in such a way as to appear to determine any
> question of
>
> (a) criminal liability on the part of a named person, or
> (b) civil liability.

It is important to appreciate that an inquest is a fact-finding enquiry
rather than a fault-finding trial, and the proceedings are inquisitorial

rather than adversarial in nature but, as the Master of the Rolls indicated giving the judgement of the court in R v North Humberside Coroner, ex parte Jamieson,[7] it is the duty of the coroner to 'ensure that the relevant facts were fully, fairly and fearlessly investigated'. The restriction in Rule 42 applies solely to the verdict, however, and, to ensure that a thorough enquiry has been conducted, there are occasions when exploration of the evidence itself must unavoidably involve matters bearing on liability.

The coroner will initially examine a witness on oath, after which relevant questions may be put to the witness by any of those with a proper interest in the proceedings, either in person or by counsel or solicitor. Those people who have this entitlement to examine witnesses are defined in Rule 20 of the Coroners Rules.

Evidence given on oath before a coroner may subsequently be used in proceedings in other courts but, as in any other court, there is a right against self-incrimination. Rule 22 provides that:

(1) no witness at an inquest shall be obliged to answer any question tending to incriminate himself, and
(2) where it appears to the coroner that a witness has been asked such a question, the coroner shall inform the witness that he may refuse to answer.

This privilege does not allow a witness to refuse to enter the witness box, and the protection against self-incrimination that it offers applies only to criminal offences, and not to possible civil or disciplinary proceedings.

If a doctor feels that his or her professional conduct may be called into question, then this should be discussed with the relevant defence organisation in good time, so that the possible need for the doctor to be legally represented can be addressed.

Inquests were held on 26,430, or just over 13 per cent, of deaths reported to coroners in 2002, continuing a reversal of the decline in inquests which had been taking place until the early 1990s.[8] The commonest verdicts were death by accident or misadventure, which was recorded in 40 per cent of cases, natural causes, recorded in 19 per cent of cases, and suicide, recorded in 14 per cent. Verdicts of death from industrial diseases almost doubled in the 10 years from 5 percent in 1984 to 1994, and this verdict was recorded in 11 percent of cases in 2002, largely reflecting the long latent period between contact with asbestos and the development of malignant mesothelioma.

Treasure trove

Apart from those duties relating to unnatural death that are provided by Section 8(1) of the Coroners Act 1988, one last vestige of the coroner's medieval duties remains. Section 30 of the Coroners Act 1988 provides that a coroner shall continue to have jurisdiction to enquire into any treasure which is found in his district, although in modern times this has more to do with the preservation of antiquities rather than for any financial benefit to the Crown. Since the first edition of this book, the Treasure Act 1996 has come into force and this has introduced new requirements for reporting and dealing with finds.

FUTURE PROPOSALS

The constraints of space in a book dealing with 'essentials' do not allow for anything other than a very brief overview of some of the proposals from the enquiries set up in the aftermath of the Shipman trial and can not, therefore, do justice to the considerable time and effort that they have spent in examining current systems for death investigation. Reading the original reports is recommended.

Both the Fundamental Review into Death Certification and Investigation[9] and the Third Report of The Shipman Inquiry (Death Certification and Investigation of Deaths by Coroners)[10] have recommended an increased level of medical input into the process of death investigation, coupled with organisational and structural reform to the service itself.

The Fundamental Review recommended that there should be a Statutory Medical Assessor in each coroner's area, who would appoint a panel of doctors to provide all community second certifications, and has recommended a regional structure to the coronership among other proposed changes. The Third Report of The Shipman Inquiry proposes an alternative structural change, creating both Judicial Coroners and Medical Coroners for each region and a radically reformed coronership which will seek to establish the cause of all deaths, supported by trained investigators.

It is not known at the present time what the final shape of the new service will be, but it remains in the general interest of the public that any deaths are investigated in a way that it is independent and thorough for the benefit of the community as a whole, while remaining sensitive to the needs, feelings and beliefs of those bereaved families most closely affected by the death.

REFERENCES AND FURTHER READING

1. The Medieval Coroner, R.F. Hunnisett, *Cambridge Studies in English Legal History*, Cambridge University Press, 1961.

Cadaveric Organs for Transplantation, A Code of Practice including the Diagnosis of Brain Death, Health Departments of Great Britain and Northern Ireland Working Party, 1983.

2. Births and Deaths Registration Act 1953.
3. Office of Population Censuses and Surveys, Completion of Medical Certificates of Cause of Death, 1990.
    Jervis on Coroners, 12 edn, Sweet and Maxwell, 2002.
4. The notes and directions accompanying books of blank Medical Certificates of Cause of Death.
5. Start RD, Delargy-Aziz Y, Dorries CP, Silocks PB, Cotton DWK. Clinicians and the Coronial system: ability of clinicians to recognise reportable deaths, *Brit. Med. J.* 1993; 306:1038–1041.
6. *R (Touche) v Inner North London Coroner*, 2001, Q.B. 1206, CA.
7. *R v North Humberside Coroner, ex parte Jamieson*, 1994, 3 W.L.R. 82, CA.
8. Statistics of Deaths Reported to Coroners: England and Wales 2002.
    The Human Tissue Act 1961.
    The Coroners Rules 1984.
    Registration of Births and Deaths Regulations 1987.
    The Coroners Act 1988.
    The Treasure Act 1996.
9. Death Certification and Investigation in England, Wales and Northern Ireland. The Report of a Fundamental Review 2003. Cm 5831.
10. The Shipman Inquiry. Third Report. Death Certification and Investigation of Deaths by Coroners. Cm 5854.

10

Tissues and organs

Sharon Korek

INTRODUCTION

Recent advances in medical technology, together with the increased use of human tissues and organs for a wide range of therapeutic treatments and research, have enhanced the potential for commercial exploitation of those tissues and organs. This has resulted in the human body, its tissues and organs being viewed from a different legal perspective. One potential change is the extent to which and in what context a proprietary status can be afforded to human tissues and organs.

The first statutory regulation of the use of the human body for dissection, teaching or research was the Anatomy Act 1832. The legislation was in part a response to the then unregulated common practice of dissecting the bodies of executed felons and paupers and served to act as a deterrent to the infamous practises of Burke and Hare, the body snatchers and grave robbers.[1] The 1832 Act together with the Anatomy Act 1871 was repealed by the Anatomy Act 1984.[2] This 1984 Act, regulates the licensing of premises where anatomy may be carried out and makes lawful the possession of anatomical specimens. It also authorises the examination of a body where an individual has requested that his body be used for anatomical examination.

Section 2 and Section 3 of the 1984 Act govern who may be in possession and carry out examinations of an 'anatomical specimen'. Such persons must keep appropriate records. Licensed individuals or teachers and students of anatomy are covered by Section 2 and Section 3. Section 4 states that the person in lawful possession may authorise the anatomical examination of the body subject to the condition that he has no reason to believe that the deceased had withdrawn his request, or that a surviving spouse or relative objects to the body being so used.

The authority under this section does not apply where an inquest or postmortem is required nor logically does it apply to persons entrusted with the body solely for the purpose of internment or cremation.

In any event the examination must be carried out within the statutory period which Section 4(10) sets at 3 years. After this period, Section 5 permits possession of the body only for the purpose of decent disposal. However, where a part of the body has been removed it may be retained for longer, under Section 5 if the identity of the person from whom it came cannot be recognised simply by examination of the part[3] and under Section 6 if the person who had donated his body also consented to the retention of removed body parts. Such continued possession is subject to the same conditions as those in Section 4. The person in possession must have been granted a licence by the Secretary of State. Failure to comply with the provisions of the Anatomy Act is a summary criminal offence punishable with a fine.[4]

CADAVERS

The Corneal Grafting Act 1952 allowed individuals to donate their eyes for medicine, but was repealed by the Human Tissue Act 1961 which governs the removal of a greater variety of parts of the body from cadavers, for medical purposes. The Human Tissue Act sets out guidance for one who 'owns' and can give consent for the use of human tissues for therapeutic use, research and transplant.

However, unlike the Anatomy Act the Human Tissue Act does not state a statutory period within which the tissue must be used. A deceased individual may by virtue of the Human Tissue Act 1961 Section 1(2) give permission for his body to be donated for therapeutic, educational and research purposes.[5] However, apart from these provisions, the deceased has few rights over the disposal of his body.

The Human Tissue Act 1961 Section 1 gives authority for the person who has legal possession of the body to give consent for the removal of parts of the body for medical purposes. Section 1(7) states that such legal possession depends on where the person is when death occurs. Hence if a person dies in hospital or in a nursing home, the person having control and management thereof has the authority to give consent for the removal of body parts.[6] However, as with the Anatomy Act, such consent is subject to the person in lawful possession making reasonable enquiry of the surviving spouse or any surviving relative and to enquire whether the deceased himself had made objections known.

At common law, it is arguable that legal possession extends to close relatives[7] for the purposes of disposal in the circumstances of them having actual possession of the body and that they would be the person(s) next entitled to be appointed as administrator of the deceased's estate.[8]

Once an individual is deceased any residual control or property rights in the body effectively cease.

FAILURE TO COMPLY WITH THE HUMAN TISSUE ACT 1961

While the Human Tissue Act 1961 sets out the criteria for the control and legal possession of a human body, unlike the Anatomy Act, arguably it provides no sanction for failure to comply.

In R v Lennox-Wright[9] the defendant falsely claimed to be a qualified doctor and gained a position at an English hospital, where he removed the eyes from a dead body for use at another hospital. He was charged contrary to Section 1(4) of the Human Tissue Act 1961, which states that *only a registered doctor can remove parts of a body*. Lennox-Wright pleaded not guilty on the grounds that the Act itself created no offence.

Despite this plea, it was held that *all* statutes that prohibit an activity create an offence at common law punishable by indictment, unless this was manifestly excluded by the statute and thus Lennox-Wright was found guilty of failing to obey a statute. This was so even though the Human Tissue Act Section 1(8) could be interpreted in such a way that the Act does not create an offence. Section 1(8) of the Act says:

> nothing in this section shall be construed as rendering unlawful any dealing with, or with any part of, the body of a deceased person which is lawful apart from this act.

At common law there is no law against removing organs from a body. Thus it is arguable that even if there is an offence of failing to obey a statute, it has no application to the Human Tissue Act. Indeed in the case of R v Horseferry Road Justices, ex p Independent Broadcasting Authority, Lloyd LJ suggested that the old doctrine of failing to obey a statute was obsolete and should be abolished.[10]

RETENTION OF HUMAN TISSUE – ALDER HEY AND BRISTOL ROYAL INFIRMARY

The legality of the retention of human tissues and organs, where the deceased's relatives were not consulted was recently the subject of much contentious and acrimonious discussion after it came to light that it was the practise at Alder Hey Children's Hospital and Bristol Royal Infirmary to remove and retain tissue and organs from the bodies of children who had died while at those hospitals. It is apparent from the Anatomy Act and Human Tissue Act that in such circumstances, the hospital would be the person in lawful possession of the body and hence have the authority to authorise the removal of tissues and organs. It is also apparent that the removal does not need the active or express consent of the relatives, but removal should be for one of the purposes set out in the Act(s). At Alder Hey and The Bristol Royal Infirmary organs had been removed during postmortem examinations and retained as a matter of routine, but not always for purposes within the Act(s).

In many cases the parent's consent was not sought or only sought in the very difficult circumstances of the parents being informed of the child's death. It was only later that parents discovered that the body of their child, which had been returned to them for the funeral, was missing an organ or in some cases several organs.

Some of the relatives have sought compensation, but such litigation is unlikely to be straightforward as the parent claimants are secondary victims and under UK law[11] such claims are subject to social and public policy control mechanisms that seek to limit the number of potential claimants.

However, it is possible that the Human Rights Act 1998 will provide a different avenue through which to pursue such claims. Article 8 of the European Convention for the Protection of Fundamental Freedoms and Human Rights is given legislative force through the Human Rights Act. Article 8 states that:

> everyone has the right to respect for his private and family life, his home and his correspondence.

It is arguable that in failing to ensure that relatives did not object to the removal and retention of tissue and organs, the NHS trusts were in breach of the rights in Article 8.

GOOD PRACTISE

While it could be said that the breaches of the Anatomy Act and Human Tissue Act in the Alder Hey and Bristol cases were minor in legal terms, they are significant in human terms.

A climate of distrust has been created between the bereaved; the clinicians and pathologists. Indeed Professor Ian Kennedy, who chaired the Bristol enquiry said of the medical profession that there was 'professional arrogance, justified when necessary by the recourse to traditional paternalism'; and in relation to the exclusion of parents from the process, that it was a 'social and ethical time bomb waiting to go off'.[12]

It is apparent that 'good practise' has not always been adhered to in the context of tissue and organ removal and retention. Some procedural improvements need to be made.

Relatives are often asked to sign consent forms, where a postmortem is to be carried out. The consent form should be reviewed so as to make it clear to relatives what tissues or organs need to be removed and retained, by whom and for what purpose. It is recognised that there is a valid need for postmortems and a need to retain tissue blocks and slides; provisions could be put in place to permit this.

The legal uncertainty that presently exists in relation to whether there is any sanction for failure to comply with the Human Tissue Act should be resolved, so as to create penalties for non-compliance.

There is another loophole that needs to be closed, that of foetuses born dead at or before 24 weeks gestation. The law does not require such births to be certified or registered. At present no legal provisions apply to the examination of such foetuses, nor to the removal and retention of tissue. It may also be recommended that clinicians and parents meet after the postmortem to discuss the outcome and where relevant receive genetic counselling or other specialist advice.

PROPERTY RIGHTS IN THE HUMAN BODY AND TISSUES

Until relatively recently, the issue of whether a human body or its tissues were property was not given much consideration or deemed to be of major significance.[13] This is primarily because while an individual might, for example, express a desire to be cremated or buried after death, in general such an individual would show little or no interest in asserting rights over any tissue that had been removed during medical treatment, in much the same way that no thought is given to the disposal of hair that is cut off by a hairdresser. If a person were to give thought to the matter, he would probably assume that the hospital would dispose of the tissue appropriately. However, with advances in medical technology and research and the concomitant opportunity for financial gain it is now necessary to consider the legal status and hence ownership of human tissue. It is increasingly likely that where such use is made of excised tissue, the individual from whom it was removed (or stolen) will make some proprietary claim to it and consequently argue a right to share in any monetary proceeds[14] or seek an injunction to prevent its use. Given the successful cloning of Dolly the sheep by Dr Ian Wilmut at the Roslyn Institute in Edinburgh in 1997 and Wilmut's assertion that cloning would soon be possible in humans,[15] then it is not surprising that there has been recent speculation that DNA 'theft' may become prevalent in a celebrity-obsessed society.[16]

THE CONCEPT OF PROPERTY

In UK law, the concept of property and property rights primarily connotes ownership and arguably all the rights that go with ownership such as the right to enjoyment, right to permit or deny access to others, right of transfer and sale.

In a number of recent cases the courts have been required to consider whether the human body or parts thereof can be categorised as property and consequently whether the rights that apply to 'real property' (land) and chattels can apply to the human body.

In R v Kelly; R v Lindsay,[17] the defendant Lindsay was a junior technician at the Royal College of Surgeons, from where he removed some thirty to forty body parts and gave them to Kelly, an artist, who wished to use the body parts as moulds for his work. Both Kelly and Lindsay were charged with theft contrary to Section 1 of the Theft Act 1968.

They argued in their defence firstly that 'parts of the body were not in law capable of being property and therefore could not be stolen' and secondly that since the Royal College of Surgeons has retained the body parts beyond the statutory period, it had no lawful possession of the parts. While the judge Rose LJ stated[18] that

> ... however questionable the origins of the principle, it has now been the common law for 150 years at least that neither a corpse, nor parts of a corpse, are in themselves and without more capable of being property protected by rights ...

he nonetheless held that

> ... once a human body or body part had undergone a process of skill by a person authorised to perform it, with the object of preserving it for the purpose of medical or scientific examination, or for the benefit of medical science, it became something quite different from an interred corpse and it thereby acquired a usefulness or value and it was capable of becoming property in the usual way, and could be stolen.

It was on this basis that Kelly and Lindsay were found guilty of theft.

Thus it would seem that organs or tissues once removed from an individual may attain the status of property by virtue of the application of some skill such as dissection or preservation technique. It was also suggested in the Kelly case that the common law does not stand still and that on some future occasion the courts may hold that human body parts are capable of being property, if they have a use beyond their mere existence.

In a recent case[19] the issue of possession took a bizarre twist when it was held that the body of a tramp, Edwin MacKenzie, which had been embalmed by an eccentric artist, Robert Lenkiewicz, was the property of the artist's estate on the basis that the artist had been asked by the tramp to embalm his body after his death and thus the artist had come lawfully into possession of the body. This raises two relevant issues. Firstly, a person can only donate his body under the Anatomy Act and Human Tissue Act for medical purposes, so has this decision created a common law right to donate a body for artistic purposes? Secondly does the concept of possession as it is used in this case, amount to property rights such that the body of MacKenzie could be put on display as part of an exhibition of Lenkiewicz's artwork.

Arguably such decisions as R v Kelly; R v Lindsay and Lenkiewicz will have a major impact on the use of human tissue for commercial purposes.

THE MOORE CASE

Property claims in relation to human tissue were discussed in the American case of Moore v Regents of the University of California.[20] Moore was undergoing treatment for hairy-cell leukaemia, in the course of which samples of blood, blood serum, skin, bone marrow aspirate and sperm were withdrawn. Moore's action was based on the fact that the defendants conducted research on his T-lymphocytes, obtained a patent on the cell-line and then shared in the considerable royalties and profits arising out of the patent. These activities were deliberately concealed from him. Moore also attempted to argue that the use of his cells amounted to the tort of conversion; a tort that protects against interference with possession and ownership interests in personal property. Moore did not succeed[21] with any of his causes of action. Panelli J said that:

> To establish a conversion, the plaintiff must establish an actual interference with his ownership or right of possession …. Where the plaintiff neither has title to the property alleged to have been converted, nor possession thereof, he cannot maintain an action in conversion.

He went on to say that:

> Since Moore clearly did not expect to retain possession of his cells following their removal, to sue for conversion he must have retained an ownership interest in them…no judicial decision supports Moore's

claim … and the subject matter of Regent's patent – the patented cell-line and the products derived from it – cannot be Moore's property.

There is no equivalent case in UK law and it remains to be seen whether in the light of the Moore case, a patient might attempt to enter into a contract with his healthcare practitioner, whereby he retained some ownership rights in his excised tissues, in the event of those tissues being commercially viable. This would be particularly pertinent where the tissue had undergone some process whereby it attained the status of property as per R v Kelly; R v Lindsay.

PROPERTY RIGHTS *IN VIVO*

Clearly, while a living person still has his organs and tissues as an integral part of his body, they are afforded some protection from abuse. The criminal law makes actual bodily harm and grievous bodily harm punishable offences by virtue of the Offences Against the Person Act 1861.[22] The civil law makes the intentional torts of trespass to the person actionable *per se*,[23] such that the wrongdoer may have to pay damages to the claimant or be subject to an injunction. Even where that person has suffered no actual harm. Indeed any medical treatment undertaken without valid consent or lawful justification may make the healthcare professional subject to civil proceedings.

Thus it could be argued that the need for consent to touching allows an individual such control over his own body as to effectively amount to the property right of being able to exclude others from access.

However, in one important respect, an individual cannot exercise property rights over his own body. The Human Organ Transplant Act 1989 Section 1 makes it an offence to 'make or receive any payment for the supply of an organ from a dead or living person'.

Similarly other rights of ownership are not absolute, a live individual cannot self-mutilate[24] or donate his heart or indeed both kidneys, even for laudable altruistic reasons where death would ensue, and in such situations the principle of the sanctity of life would prevail and thus trump an individual's rights 'to do as he pleased' with his 'property'. Even where organs or tissues have been donated within the confines of the law,[25] the donor has little control over subsequent use.[26]

In other ways, rights that would conform to the concept of 'property' are denied in the context of the human body, or overridden, such as when an individual is lawfully detained under the Mental Health Act 1983 or when a coroner requires a postmortem examination under the Coroners Act 1988. The justification for this approach is arguably based in public policy.

Thus it is clear that while it is the case that a living individual has such rights in his own body that would afford respect for his autonomy and would even extend to a due regard for confidentiality, these rights would not amount to full property rights such as those given to 'real property' (land) or chattels.

GAMETES AND EMBRYOS

The donation, use and storage of gametes and embryos is regulated by the Human Fertilisation and Embryology Act 1990, which restricts the activities it regulates to licensed premises and to those who have been granted a licence. All licensed activities are overseen by the Human Fertilisation and Embryology Authority, which are established by Section 5 of the Act.

Most of the licensed activities relate to the provision of fertility treatment, but licences can be obtained for treatment; storage and research as set out in Schedule 2 of the Act and including 'increasing knowledge about the causes of congenital disease; developing more effective contraception and developing methods for detecting the presence of gene or chromosome abnormalities in embryos before implantation'. Arguably, it is within the context of such investigations that the potential for commercial exploitation becomes apparent and consequently the issue of ownership becomes relevant.

Schedule 3 of the Act specifies that consent for the use of gametes must be given in writing by the person who donates the gametes or in the case of embryos, by both parties who contributed to its creation.

Schedule 3 Section 4(2) does not allow the consent to be varied once the gametes or embryos have been used for the purposes of research or fertility treatment. While this section of the Act may not have been written with commercial gain and property rights in mind, the effect of the section is to prevent an individual from exercising any property rights in his or her gametes and embryos by making it impossible to reclaim them, should the research that utilised them prove to be commercially viable.

To argue that sperm cannot be property would seem to be a contradictory statement, when it is well known that a man may sell his sperm, but if such a sale relates to the 'service' of providing the sperm rather than the sperm itself, the contradiction is rationalised. The non-property approach to sperm and embryos is consistently applied in other areas of UK law. For example, 'sale' is made unlawful in the context of surrogacy arrangements.[27]

A similar attitude has been adopted by the French courts. In the case of Parpalaix v CECOS[28] the court refused to recognise any property interest in sperm. However, this approach is not universally applied in other jurisdictions. In California the Court of Appeal held in Hecht v Kane[29] that a deceased man who had previously consented to the use, by his partner, of his sperm, had an interest in the sperm amounting to 'property' within the meaning of the Probate Code. The German Bundesgerichtshof[30] has ruled that normal rules of personal property apply not only to stored sperm but to transplant organs as well.

CONCLUSION

Thus it would seem that the concept of property as applied to the human body, its tissues and organs has a variable definition according to which organ or tissue it is applied to and the intended use of that tissue or organ.

It is arguable that it is now time to rethink and rationalise this ambivalent attitude to property rights in human organs and tissues. This is particularly so when it is apparent that an individual from whom tissue is removed is denied any property rights in that tissue, but any third party who then uses or changes that tissue in some way can not only gain property rights in that organ or tissue but can then go on to protect that interest through the law of patents. Indeed the biotechnology industry is encouraged in commercial profit making activities on the basis that everyone benefits from the development of new therapeutic treatments and remedies for diseases.

A balance needs to be struck so that, the fundamental relationship an individual has with his own body and his right to control it and arguably profit from it, can be reconciled with the commercial use of his body by others.

The need for clarification of ownership rights in human tissue may become acute in the context of the commodification of an individual's DNA, particularly in the circumstances of an individual's DNA being taken without his knowledge.

REFERENCES AND NOTES

1. Burke was a notorious murderer and he was executed in 1829. His exploits were so infamous that the phrase 'to be Burked' found its way into *The Shorter Oxford English Dictionary* (1st edn, 1933).

2. The 1984 Act came into force in February 1988.
3. Thus a head could not be retained and arguably neither could an arm that had a distinctive tattoo.
4. S11(5), (7), (8) and Reg. 5.
5. A body may also be donated under the Anatomy Act 1984, but this is limited to dissection for the purpose of studying morphology (S1(4)). Further, the Human Tissue Act 1961 S1(5) gives this Act precedence over the Anatomy Act.
6. The Transplant of Human Organs Bill 2001 sought to change the wording of S1(7) so as to substitute 'Health Authority of NHS Trust' for 'person lawfully'. The Bill was not passed before the dissolution of Parliament and so did not take effect.
7. R v Gwynedd County Council, *ex parte* B (1991) 7 BMLR 120 CA in which it was held that the parent of an unmarried child had the right to possess and dispose of the body. The issue of who had the right to possession of a deceased child's body arose out of an appeal by foster parents for judicial review of the decision that the natural mother of the child, which had been in care, had the right and duty to bury the child. It was held that a council's parental rights and duties with respect to a child in its care under s2 Child Care Act 1980 ceased on the child's death and any parental right or duty to bury the child reverts to the natural parents.
8. Non-Contentious Probate Rules 1987 (SI 1987 No 2024), rule 22.
9. *R v Lennox-Wright*, 1973, *Crim LR*, 529 (CCC).
10. *R v Horseferry Road Justices, ex parte* Independent Broadcasting Authority, 1987, QB 54; 1986, 2 ALL ER 666 (Div Ct).
11. *White & Ors (Respondents) v Chief Constable of South Yorks & Ors (Appellants) sub nom Frost & Ors v CCSY* 1999 HL 1 ALL ER 1.
12. Organ Retention Scandals, Dr Peter Ellis. 2001, J.P.I.L Issue 3/01.
13. The Nuffield Council on Bioethics discussed the issue of property rights in human bodies and tissues in its report: *Human Tissue: Ethical and Legal Issues*, 1995.
14. *Moore v Regents of the University of California*, 1990, 793 P 2d 479 (Cal Sup Ct).
15. *The Times*, 7 March 1997.
16. Gary Slapper, writing in The Times said that The Human Genetics Commission will soon ask ministers to consider criminalizing the theft of DNA material... particularly at risk are celebrities. Deterrent to DNA Hunters. *The Times*, 19 March 2002.
17. 1998, 3 ALL ER 741.
18. *Ibid.* at 749.
19. *The Times*, 12 November 2002.
20. *Moore v Regents of the University of California* (1990) S1 Cal 3d 120 (Cal Sup Ct); (1990), 793 P2d 479 (Cal Sup Ct).
21. The majority remanded the case for trial on the issue of whether Moore had given any valid consent for his cells to be used for research. The issue revolved around the fiduciary duty owed to Moore by the doctors to disclose any conflicts of interest that might affect their medical judgement.
22. Offences Against Person Act 1865 S18; S20.
23. Actionable *per se* means actionable without the need for the claimant to prove that they have suffered any harm.

24. *R v Brown*, 1993, 2 ALL ER 75, HL.
25. Human Organ Transplant Act 1989; Unrelated Live Transplant Regulatory Authority, ULTRA; Human Tissue Act 1961.
26. An Investigation into Conditional Organ Donation 2000 (www.doh.gov.uk/pub/docs/doh/organdonation.pdf) was set up by the government to investigate conditional donation of organs. It reached the conclusion that organs should not be accepted by the UK Transplant Support Service Authority (UKTSSA) where there were racist preconditions as this would breach S20(1) and S31(1) of the Race Relations Act 1976 and as such would be unlawful.
27. Surrogacy Arrangements Act 1985 S2.
28. Journal of Clinical Pathology 1984.II.20321.
29. 16 Cal App 4th 836 (1993).
30. Bundesgerichtshof, 9 Nov 1993, BGHZ, 124, 52.

11

Organ donation

Sue Sutherland

INTRODUCTION

Transplantation of organs and tissues became a recognised therapeutic intervention during the 20th century. The first cornea transplant took place in 1905, followed by the first kidney in 1954, liver in 1963 and heart in 1967.

Over the years transplantation has become easier and safer and it is now possible to transplant kidneys, heart and the heart valves, lungs, pancreas, liver and small bowel, corneas, bone, tendons and skin. All forms of transplants are carried out in the UK and the outcomes for patients in terms of their own survival and that of the transplant are amongst the best in the world. Transplantation is now recognised as the treatment of choice for people with organ failure and an increasing number of people could have their lives saved or improved by a transplant. Indeed for end stage liver, heart and lung failure there is no alternative to transplantation. Those in renal failure can be maintained on dialysis but their life expectancy is better if they are transplanted.[1] The demand for organs is high and is likely to increase in the foreseeable future as kidney and liver disease becomes more prevalent in the population and until biological and technological solutions become feasible. For over a decade the supply of human donor organs has not matched the demand (Figure 11.1) and in 2002, 400 people who were on the UK waiting list for an organ transplant died before an organ could be found for them. In addition many more will die before they get the opportunity to be listed on the national transplant waiting list.

During 2001 the world's leading transplant centres carried out 23,000 kidney transplants from cadaveric donors, 8,200 kidney transplants from live donors, 11,000 liver transplants and 4,600 heart and heart/lung transplants. The same countries recorded the deaths of 2,800 people who died while on the waiting list.[2] The last decade has seen an increase in kidney transplants largely due to donation from live donors, an increase in liver transplants due to the skill of surgeons being able to split cadaveric donor

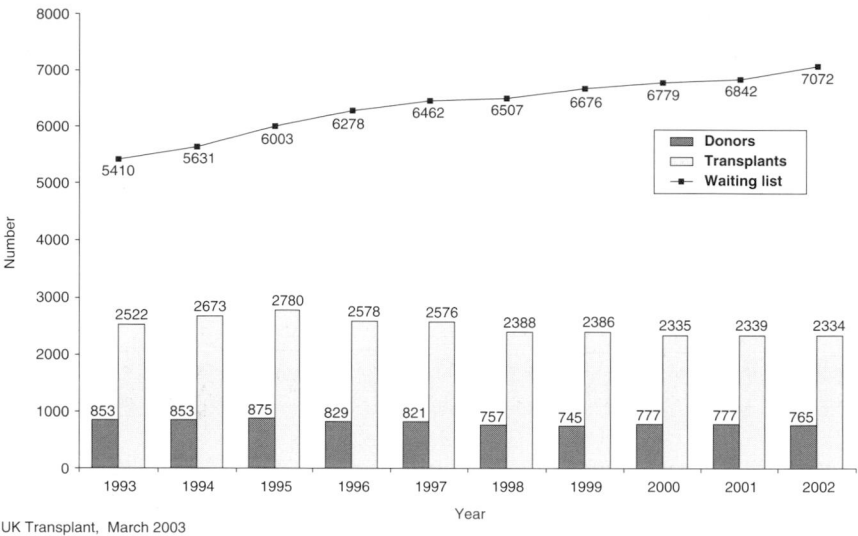

UK Transplant, March 2003

Figure 11.1 Numbers of cadaveric donors and transplants in the UK 1993–2002, and patients on the active and suspended waiting lists on 31st December.

livers and a negligible increase in the numbers of heart and heart–lung transplants due to the chronic shortage of heart-beating cadaveric donors. Supply has not been able to keep pace with increasing demand and the situation in the UK is consistent with the international picture.

From the 1960s onwards it became apparent that in order to ensure that scarce organs were used to maximum benefit there needed to be national arrangements for organ donation and allocation. This would ensure that people regardless of their domicile would receive an organ based on their clinical need and characteristics.

Organ donation and allocation is the responsibility of an National Health Service (NHS) Special Health Authority, UK Transplant, and a service is provided to all countries within the UK. These national sharing arrangements have been maintained and encouraged through the devolution of power and each country of the UK actively supports and funds organ donation and allocation to be maintained on a UK wide basis.

UK Transplant holds a national waiting list of those waiting for transplant and matches and allocates organs as they become available. As allocation is based on clinical characteristics such as tissue type, there can be no direct discrimination in relation to ethnicity, gender, etc. However increasingly people from non-white ethnic groups are disadvantaged indirectly for two reasons. Firstly renal failure is more prevalent in their group and secondly they are less likely to be organ donors, making fewer organs with appropriate tissue type available. The consequence is that these people are forming a greater proportion of the national transplant waiting list for kidney transplants.[3]

The UK also participates in organ exchange arrangements with other European countries to ensure that organs that cannot be used in the originating country are offered to other countries and not wasted. This works well on the basis that the larger the donor pool the more likelihood of getting a match for patients with rare features (e.g. very small child).

Heart, lung and liver transplantation is commissioned on a national basis from 6 adult and 1 paediatric heart transplant centres and 7 liver transplant centres. Kidney transplantation is commissioned locally by primary care Trusts from 24 kidney transplant centres. Cornea transplants are not commissioned separately from other ophthalmic procedures and are carried out in many ophthalmic departments in hospitals across the country.

LEGISLATION

The first Anatomy Act was passed in 1832 following the Burke and Hare scandal involving the sale of suffocated bodies. Since then legislation and guidance on the use of human organs and tissue has grown in a piece-meal fashion, sometimes in response to scandals (see also Chapter 10).

There are currently two key pieces of legislation governing organ donation and transplantation in the UK, the Human Tissue Act 1961[4] and the Human Organ Transplants Act 1989.[5] The Human Tissue Act in particular is widely regarded as unsatisfactory and in need of reform. It is currently based on the need for individuals to 'opt in' to organ donation. In response to the Alder Hey organ retention scandal, not a transplant scandal, the Government has recently consulted on organ and tissue donation through a document entitled 'Human bodies–Human choices'[6] in order to consider a more comprehensive and coherent legal framework and this may lead to legislative changes during 2003–2004.

Furthermore in 2000 the Human Rights Act 1998 came into force and incorporated the European Convention on Human Rights into domestic law. As yet the courts have not considered the implications for existing law on the removal, retention and use of organs and tissue. There are a number of Articles that could be considered as applicable to organ donation. For example Article 2 gives a right to life and it could be argued that governments should do more to make organs available to those who would otherwise die without them. Government could consider including an 'opt out' arrangement that assumed that in appropriate circumstances people would be expected to donate their organs on death unless there was an individual expression to the contrary. Article 12 gives the right to marry and found a family. Women with renal failure are unlikely to have a successful pregnancy. Again what steps should a government take to ensure they receive a kidney transplant in order that they can have a family?

THE HUMAN TISSUE ACT 1961

The Human Tissue Act as originally enacted consisted of four sections only two of which concern the removal and use of organs and tissue. Its purpose is as follows:

> to make provision with respect to the use of bodies of the deceased persons for therapeutic purposes and purposes of medical education and research and with respect to the circumstances in which post mortem examinations are carried out and to permit the cremation of bodies removed for anatomical examination

The Act states (Section 1) that if a person has expressed a wish in writing, or orally in the presence of two or more witnesses, that their body or any specified part may be used for therapeutic purposes after their death, the person lawfully in possession of the body may, unless there is reason to believe that the request was subsequently withdrawn, authorise removal from the body any part in accordance with the request.

If there is no evidence of such a wish, the person lawfully in charge of the body of the deceased person may authorise the removal of any part of body provided that, if having made such reasonable enquiries as may be practicable, there is no reason to believe that the deceased had expressed an objection to their body being so dealt with after their death and had not withdrawn it, or that the surviving spouse or any surviving relative of the deceased objects to the body being so dealt with.

THE HUMAN ORGANS TRANSPLANTS ACT 1989

The Human Organ Transplants Act 1989 was introduced in direct response to the 'kidneys for sale' scandal which exposed an international trade in human organs.

It is an Act to prohibit commercial dealings in human organs intended for transplanting and to control the transplanting of such organs between persons who are not genetically related.

It is also an offence to advertise the buying or selling of organs or to withhold information required by law about transplant operations. The Act also made it illegal to transplant an organ removed from a living person unless the donor and recipient were genetically related or unless approval was given by Unrelated Live Transplant Regulatory Authority (ULTRA), the guidance for which is contained in the Human Organ Transplants (unrelated persons) Regulations 1989[7] which allows donation between genetically unrelated donors and recipients (e.g. husband and wife, partners, etc.).

The practical application of this act is that registered medical practitioners will be expected, by the completion of written information, to account for all organs that they have either removed and/or transplanted. UK Transplant monitors compliance with the Act on behalf of the UK Governments.

The Human Organ Transplants Act currently provides a range of penalties for non-compliance from fines for failing to provide information to a maximum of 3 months in prison for commercial dealing in organs or transplanting persons not genetically related without approval.

NHS ORGAN DONOR REGISTER

The Human Tissue Act relies on individuals to 'opt in' to organ donation during their life so their wishes are known on their death. In the past those opting in would have made their wishes known to relatives and perhaps carried an organ donor card. More recently in 1994 the UK established an organ donor register run and administered by UK Transplant which records the wishes of those people who wish to donate organs and tissue on their death. Individuals can sign on to the register through a number of routes. They can sign on to the register when they register with a General Practitioner, when they apply for a driving licene or passport and, in some areas, when they complete their electoral roll information. The register currently contains the names of 10.5 million people and it is the Government's intention that it should have 16 million names on it by 2010.

The information on the register can be made available to designated staff in the NHS who wish to ascertain the wishes of a deceased person. It is widely accepted that when relatives know that their loved one wanted to donate they are unlikely to object.

In a recent public attitude survey[8] 90% of respondents said they were in favour of organ donation in principle and therefore it is imperative, while opt in legislation is in place, that more people are encouraged to make their wishes known on the register.

The vast majority of countries in Europe, as well as the USA and Canada, also maintain organ donor registers. Some of those registers support opt out legislation where it is accepted that in appropriate situations organs will be removed for transplantation unless the deceased had made a written expression to the contrary.

DONORS OF ORGANS

Organs can be donated in both life (living) and after death (cadaveric). After death and in appropriate circumstances a donor may be able to donate all major organs, corneas and tissue. A live donor can normally donate one kidney, a segment of liver or a piece of lung.

There are two types of cadaveric donor, heart-beating and non-heart-beating. In the former the person's death is diagnosed following brain stem death tests and in the latter when their heartbeat has irreversibly ceased. Heart-beating donors are treated on a ventilator and as a result their circulation is maintained and they can be considered for multi-organ donation. Non-heart-beating donors can be considered for kidney and liver donation but the early perfusion of these organs is necessary to preserve them for transplantation.

Although the Human Tissue Act only requires that reasonable enquiries be made of relatives to establish that the deceased had not expressed an objection to organ donation, it has become standard practice to seek the consent of relatives for donation. In gaining consent transplant co-ordinators take a detailed clinical history to guard against the transfer of transmissible disease between donor and recipient. While the detailed clinical history of a donor is essential, the practice of gaining consent is questionable and in public attitude research carried out in 2002[8], 61% of respondents agreed that it should not be necessary to get further permission from the next of kin when the individual had confirmed their wish to donate on death by opting in.

DEFINITION OF DEATH

There is no statutory definition of death enshrined in UK law. Death is a process not an event and is diagnosed by the irreversible cessation of respiration and heart beat or the irreversible cessation of brain stem function. In those who are potential organ donors, doctors who are not part of the transplant team diagnose death. A Code of Practice[9] has been drawn up by an expert working group on behalf of the UK health departments and which includes the diagnosis of death by brain stem tests.

INCREASING THE NUMBERS OF DONORS AND THE UK MODEL OF ORGAN DONATION

At the end of the 1990s, Ministers in the UK became concerned about the decline in the number of organs available for transplantation and the decreasing number of transplants being undertaken (Figure 11.1). The UK performance is significantly worse than most other European countries as shown in Table 11.1.

This performance is despite an audit of deaths in intensive care units during 1989 and 1990 that confirmed that out of a total of 24,023 deaths, 3,266 patients had a diagnosis of brain stem death but only 1,232 became donors. The study confirmed that there is potential for more organ donation if the systems were in place and working efficiently.

In response to falling solid organ and cornea donation rates, the UK governments gave UK Transplant a wider remit enshrined in legislation to include improving organ donation rates. In 2002 a UK model for organ donation was implemented as follows:

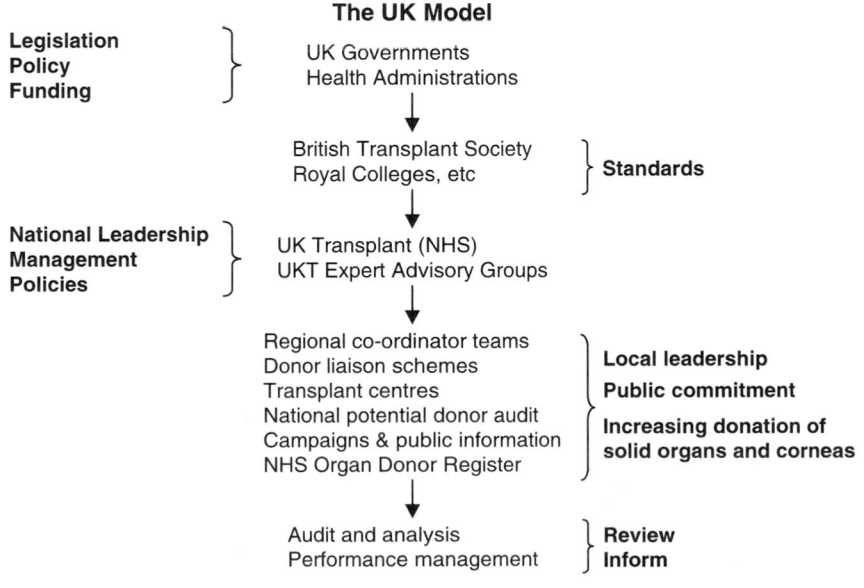

Table 11.1 Organ donation and transplant activity per million population (pmp) in Europe, 2001.

	Euro-transplant[1]	France	Italy	Spain	Scandia transplant[2]	UK[3]	ROI[3]
Cadaveric donors	1701	1066	988	1335	331	777	68
pmp	**14.3**	**17.8**	**17.1**	**32.5**	**13.8**	**13.1**	**18.2**
Cadaveric kidney transplants	3077	1921	1447	1893	599	1385	122
pmp	**25.9**	**32.0**	**25.0**	**46.1**	**25.0**	**23.4**	**32.6**
Living donor kidney transplants	610	101	99	31	249	358	2
pmp	**5.1**	**1.7**	**1.7**	**0.8**	**10.4**	**6.1**	**0.5**
Liver transplants	1316	859	831	1004	217	684	35
pmp	**11.1**	**14.3**	**14.4**	**24.4**	**9.0**	**11.6**	**9.4**
Heart + heart/lung transplants	600	342	316	341	98	204	11
pmp	**5.0**	**5.7**	**5.5**	**8.3**	**4.1**	**3.4**	**2.9**
Lung transplants	269	117	62	143	67	93	–
pmp	**2.3**	**1.9**	**1.1**	**3.5**	**2.8**	**1.6**	–

[1] Eurotransplant includes Germany, Austria, Belgium, Luxembourg, The Netherlands and Slovenia.
[2] Scandia Transplant includes Denmark, Norway, Finland and Sweden.
[3] Figures taken from National Transplant Database, February 2002. All others are provisional figures from Organizacion Nacional de Trasplantes (ONT).
Note: Definitions of a cadaveric solid organ donor vary between countries.

The key elements of the UK model include the need for a clear legislative framework as described previously and government support. All countries in the UK are committed to improving transplant rates and endorse the need for the UK to work together, collectively, on organ donation. The Governments are producing or have produced policy documents, e.g. the Transplant Plans, National Service Frameworks etc. which emphasise this commitment and specify the standards and quantity of service that patients can expect.

All countries in the UK express their commitment by providing specific funding for the purpose of supporting a national organ sharing service and increasing organ donation rates.

National leadership and co-ordination of the service is provided by UK Transplant who are supported by expert advisory groups who are representative of all professional staff involved in organ and cornea transplantation in the UK and patients and donor families.

Across the country regional teams of transplant co-ordinators are in place to lead and co-ordinate the service at local level. Donor liaison doctors and nurses in intensive care services assist by ensuring that all potential donors are identified and their wishes about donation ascertained.

A national transplant database is maintained and collects data on all donors and transplants. Follow-up information on people who have been transplanted is collected until their graft fails or they die so that national analysis can provide an evidence base for changing practice. The analysis of this data since the early 1970s has contributed to UK patient and graft survival rates that are among the best in the world.

THE FUTURE

In 2002–2003 transplant rates using cadaveric organs in the UK rose significantly for the first time in a number of years. This is most likely to be due to the implementation of the UK model described previously and is significant given that death rates in the UK have fallen by 20% in the last decade[10] and continue to fall making less donors available.

From 2003–2004 the UK will be the first country in the world to publish the results of a continuous potential donor audit that will quantify the actual numbers of people who are dying in circumstances that make it possible for them to be considered for solid organ donation. This will confirm whether or not the supply of human organs in the UK can ever meet the demand. In the meantime and until alternative technological and biological solutions become feasible, future success is dependant on continued Government and public support and a National Health

Service that has the infrastructure to ensure that facilities are available to care for potential donors and the recipients of the precious gift of a donated organ.

REFERENCES AND FURTHER READING

1. Comparison of Mortality in patients listed for renal transplant: reduced risk for transplantation vs dialysis, British Transplantation Society Annual Congress Meeting 2002.
2. International figures on organ donation and transplantation 2001 – Committee of experts on the organisational aspects of co-operation in organ transplantation
3. UK Transplant Activity Report 2001.
4. The Human Tissue Act 1961.
5. Human Organ Transplant Act 1989.
6. Human Bodies – Human Choices, DoH 2002.
7. Human Organ Transplants (Unrelated Persons) Regulations 1989.
8. Barriers to Joining the Organ Donor Register. RBA Research Jan 2003.
9. Cadaveric organs for transplantation – A Code of Practice including diagnosis of brain death – Health Departments of Great Britain and Northern Ireland 1998.
10. Office for National Statistics.

12

Living wills

Sharon Korek

INTRODUCTION

Living wills, also known as Advance Directives, allow an individual to participate in future decisions about his healthcare provision. The Advance Directive is written at a time when that individual is in 'good' mental and physical health, in anticipation of a future event that deprives him of his autonomy and decision making capacity.[1]

THE ROLE AND SCOPE OF LIVING WILLS

Living wills may take the form of an instruction that specifies consent to lifesaving resuscitation and treatment, or one which specifies refusal of consent, which would lead to withdrawal or withholding of life saving treatment. In either case the instruction cannot amount to what would be directions for euthanasia, which remains illegal. Living wills are also quite distinct from and should not be confused with cases such as that of Diane Pretty[2] which concern voluntary euthanasia or assisted suicide.

Prior discussions between an individual and his healthcare professional that form the basis of a living will, represent the exercise of 'actual' autonomy by that individual. However at the point at which the living will would be put into effect, the individual cannot participate and hence there is a lack of contemporaneous personal choice. The contemporaneous nature of any decision is a significant factor in deciding whether a living will should be followed or not, particularly when the patient's instructions would lead inevitably to his death. While there is no set format[3] for a living will, the instructions must be very clear if they are to be followed as it is possible that an individual, when faced with the actuality of his predicament, might change his mind, or the living will may not have envisaged the precise circumstances the patient finds himself in.

Such a situation may arise in the course of a disease that is gradually debilitating. In the earlier stages of the disease, healthcare professionals may be reluctant to withdraw treatment particularly where advances in medical technology may change the prognosis. In such situations, a pertinent factor in determining whether the living will was a current representation of the patient's wishes would depend on how recently the living will had been written and perhaps the extent to which the healthcare professional had participated in formulating the content.

A clarification must be made as to what constitutes consent to treatment. While an individual may request or give consent to resuscitation and treatment he cannot demand it. Healthcare professionals cannot be compelled[4] by law or their own professional guidelines to carry out procedures which they judge to be clinically inappropriate, futile or of no benefit to the patient.[5] In Re J[6] Lord Donaldson MR said

> No one can dictate the treatment to be given … neither the court, parents nor doctors. There are checks and balances. The doctors can recommend treatment A in preference to treatment B. They can also refuse to adopt treatment C on the grounds that it is medically contra-indicated or for some other reason is a treatment which they could not conscientiously administer. The court or parents for their part can refuse to consent to treatment A or B or both, but cannot insist on C … .[7]

In Re R, Lord Donaldson referred to consent as being

> merely a key which unlocks the door … the decision to treat is dependent upon an exercise of his own [the health carer's] professional judgement …[8]

Thus a living will can do no more than indicate a patient's anticipated treatment preferences.

SELF OWNERSHIP

Self ownership or the right to determine what is done with one's own body, finds its expression in the ethical concept of self-determination or autonomy. Autonomy respects the principle of bodily integrity; it is the concept that every person has the right to have his bodily integrity protected against invasion by others. It may also be described as the personal rule of self that is free from both controlling interferences by others and from personal limitations that prevent meaningful choice, such as inadequate understanding. The concept of autonomy has long been recognised and upheld by the common law and has gained in significance since the late 1950s and it could be said that it now pervades the whole of medical practice.[9] Indeed the law permits few exceptions to the principle of self-determination, subject to the *de minimis* principle.[10] Thus any touching without consent may lead to an action in battery. The cause of action arises not from the degree of harm suffered but from the affront to bodily integrity and thus is actionable *per se*.[11] In Re T Lord Donaldson cited Robins JA in Malette v Shulman[12] and said

> The right to determine what shall be done with one's own body is a fundamental right in our society. The concepts inherent in this right are the bedrock upon which the principles of self-determination and individual autonomy are based. Free individual choice in matters affecting this right should, in my opinion, be accorded very high priority

This is so even where the refusal to consent may be seen by others to be irrational, repugnant or morally questionable.[13] This approach is similar to jurisprudence in other parts of the world. In Cruzan v Director, Missouri Department of Health,[14] the US Supreme Court said

> No right is held more sacred, or is more carefully guarded ... than the right of every individual to the possession and control of his own person, free from all restraint or interference of others, unless by clear and unquestionable authority of law.

US law recognises a much stronger doctrine of informed consent. However, the doctrine of informed consent is not recognised in UK Law in the same way that it is in the US. In the US the doctrine of informed consent relates to the amount of information that a patient should be given about proposed treatment options, in addition to the information which is given, so as to obtain the patient's consent and thereby avoid an action in negligence or the tort of battery. Whereas in the UK, there is merely a requirement that the patient be informed in broad terms, of the nature of the proposed treatment.

It is arguable that cases such as Re S[15] demonstrate a marked shift towards judicial respect for self-determination and away from paternalism. Today this approach is particularly relevant in the context of living wills where it can perform the role of preventing the 'doctor knows best' paternalistic attitude to crucial decision-making. This is even more so where it is accepted that the decision to consent or refuse to consent is a quality of life choice rather than a medical decision.

Where a patient is unconscious or incapable of giving consent, a doctor may treat provided that he does so, out of necessity, in the best interests of the patient so as to save the patient's life or restore him to a state where he regains competency to consent or refuse. Clearly this exception, or justification to treat without consent cannot operate in the face of a living will, the instructions in which clearly refuse such intervention. This is in line with existing common law.[16]

Hence when the instructions within a living will are honoured, it shows a regard for that individual's self-determination, because it respects that individual's subjective view of what quality of life is acceptable for himself. However, the situation may arise where a patient who while competent did not make a living will or give any anticipatory instructions as to his wishes in the event of becoming incompetent. The principle of self-determination still persists in such circumstances and is still deserving of respect. Hence the courts are put in the difficult position of determining the lawfulness of continued treatment or medical intervention. This issue was considered in Bland[17] and more recently by Dame Butler Sloss in the case of Ms B.[18]

INFORMED REFUSAL

It is arguable that consent and refusal to medical treatment should be given equal respect, where the patient has the capacity to make decisions. However, it is apparent from case law that this is not always so.[19] This discrepancy relates to the fact that a patient who consents is agreeing with medical opinion as to what is in his 'best interests', but in refusing, is rejecting the greater medical knowledge and years of training and experience of the healthcare professional. Such refusal could also be said to challenge the most fundamental of principles, that of the sanctity of human life.[20] Thus it would seem that greater capacity is required of a patient to refuse than to consent. This approach was apparent in the case of Re MB,[21] where a pregnant woman who refused a caesarean section was considered by the court to be incompetent on the basis that she had a needle phobia. However, when she later changed her mind and consented, she was suddenly deemed to have sufficient capacity to do so.

In either context, a patient needs to have sufficient information on which to base his decision. The healthcare professional should disclose information beyond that minimal level required to avoid a claim for battery.[22] However, not all decisions taken in a healthcare context are medical in nature and thus where there is a living will, it could be said that the decision to consent or refuse is not a medical one, but rather a life choice, quality of life decision and on this basis the patient's views should take precedence over those of the doctor.

CURRENT STATUS

> It is uncertain whether healthcare personnel are required to carry out the terms of a living will: conversely, those who, in good faith, act in accordance with living wills are not assured immunity from civil or criminal prosecution. No penalties are provided for the destruction, concealment, forgery or other misuse of living wills which leaves them somewhat vulnerable to abuse[23]

While this quote is from the USA, similar uncertainties would seem to persist in the UK.

The legal status of living wills has not as yet been tested in UK courts, but it seems that in clear cases they will be enforceable. Where the courts have been required to discuss similar issues, such as the withdrawal of food and hydration from a persistent vegetative state (PVS) patient[24] and cessation of artificial ventilation[25] their Lordships have found in favour of recognising the right to refuse life supporting treatment. In Re T[26] the Court considered, obiter, the validity of a patient's anticipatory refusal of treatment. While the court avoided giving effect to the patient's wishes on the grounds that her refusal was vitiated by her mother's undue influence, it nonetheless recognised the legal effect of a 'properly' made anticipatory refusal. This view was supported in Bland[27] despite the fact that Bland had not in fact given any anticipatory instructions. Lord Keith said[28]

> Such a person is completely at liberty to decline to undergo treatment, even if the result of his doing so will be that he will die. This extends to the situation where the person, in anticipation of this, through one cause or another, entering into a condition such as PVS, gives clear instructions that in such event he is not to be given medical care, including artificial feeding, designed to keep him alive

However, in the recent case of Ms B,[29] the patient had made a living will and when she later became tetraplegic she sought to rely on the existence of the living will when she told her doctors that she no longer wished to be ventilated. The doctors informed her that the terms of the living will were not specific enough to authorise withdrawal of ventilation. The court held that in such circumstances the NHS Trust Hospital should not hesitate to make an application to the High Court or seek advice from the Official Solicitor. While in the case of Ms B the court recognised the right of the (competent) patient to withdraw her consent to treatment at any time in the future, if and when she should so decide, it did not make any ruling as to the legal status of her living will. Instead it relied on her verbal testimony as to her wishes for her future and in so doing sought to determine her competence and capacity to reach such a decision.

Thus it would seem that the status of living wills is derived not from any inherent value or quality they may have, but from a patient's pre-existing right, ingrained in the common law and human rights law, to consent to or refuse treatment, even where death might result. The patient may decide to use the vehicle of a living will to make known his consent or refusal. But it is arguable that this alone, in the absence of any other evidence and particularly where the patient is unable to affirm the living will, will not be sufficient for healthcare professionals to rely on without more, unless it is unequivocal and precise and in anticipation of the exact predicament that the patient finds himself in. Lord Goff [30] said

> … though in such circumstances special care may be necessary to ensure that the prior refusal of consent is still properly to be regarded as applicable in the circumstances which have subsequently occurred

In Re C[31] an elderly chronic schizophrenic refused to permit the amputation of his foot that had become gangrenous, unless he gave his written consent. Despite the clarity of the patient's wishes, the doctors sought a declaration from the court. The court granted an injunction preventing the amputation and so upheld the patient's advance directive.

Healthcare professionals who find themselves faced with a refusal of treatment in the form of a living will may prefer a declaration from the court, as to the validity of the living will and the lawfulness of the cessation of life saving treatment, as only this would give them immunity from prosecution. Indeed the Law Commission[32] recommends that a living will should not preclude the provision of 'basic care', namely care to maintain bodily cleanliness and to alleviate severe pain, as well as the provision of direct oral nutrition and hydration. Hence healthcare professionals should not be obliged to follow living wills that purport to refuse this level of care.

Despite the recognition of the significance of living wills in the recent case of Re AK,[33] in which a 19-year old was ventilator-dependant and could only communicate by blinking his eyes, healthcare professionals remain cautious in their reliance on living wills. In a recent poll of 300 UK doctors, 96% accepted the right of the competent patient to refuse treatment, but only 61% were prepared to end a patient's treatment knowing that death would result.[34]

It is perhaps also worthy of note that the question of whether a refusal of life sustaining treatment constitutes suicide, is not as yet resolved, as are the insurance implications of a patient having died as a result of a doctor withholding treatment in accordance with a living will.

CRITERIA FOR A LIVING WILL

The criteria for a living will are not dissimilar to those required for valid consent or refusal for imminent medical treatment. For a valid refusal the patient must be (a) competent at the time the decision was made, (b) free from undue influence, (c) sufficiently informed and (d) the patient must intend his refusal to apply to the circumstances which arise.

A patient's competence and freedom from undue influence raise no particular problems in the context of living wills. However, it is arguable that the amount of information a patient needs to make a valid anticipatory refusal is greater than it would be for a refusal for an immediate treatment choice, in that he should be aware of the nature and effect of the procedure he is refusing and whether any alternative treatments exist.

It is the last of the criteria mentioned above that requires particular comment. This criterion may permit the court to decline to follow the instructions in a living will, on the basis that the patient had not anticipated the actual predicament in which he finds himself. This would permit the court to undermine its apparent commitment to a patient's right to self-determination. Indeed the doctors declined to follow the living will made by Ms B (ante) as it had not addressed her precise predicament.

HEALTHCARE PROXY

In the absence of a validly appointed healthcare proxy or surrogate decision maker, no one has the right to consent or refuse on behalf of an incompetent adult.[35] A healthcare proxy may tell the doctor what the patient's instructions are, but no legal power is transferred to such a proxy to take the decision on the patient's behalf. Such a proxy is not to be confused with powers of attorney granted under the Enduring Powers of Attorney Act 1985, which cover decisions restricted to the 'property and other affairs' of an individual.

The Mental Health Act 1983 Section 7 allows for the appointment of a guardian, but such a person does not have the power to consent to treatment.[36] (see also Chapter 8) While a doctor may discuss matters with a relative or next of kin, and a court may give the views and opinions of relatives due consideration, such views and opinions have no legal standing. In Re T[37] Lord Donaldson MR unequivocally stated the position in the UK

> There seems to be the view in the medical profession that in such emergency circumstances the next of kin should be asked to consent on behalf of the patient and that if possible, treatment should be postponed until that consent has been obtained. This is a misconception because the next of kin has no legal right to consent or to refuse consent

In Cruzan[38] it was argued that the choice between life and death is a deeply personal one and not all incompetent patients have loved ones available to serve as surrogate decision makers. Even if they do, the state is entitled to guard against potential abuses in such situations. The family may make a mistake and misjudge the patient's wishes and there is no automatic assurance that the views of close family members will be the same as those of the patient.

Indeed even the court has no absolute jurisdiction in such matters. In Re F[39] it was held that its *parens patriae* jurisdiction did not apply to adults, even if the adult was incompetent. This position has arisen because when the Mental Health Act 1959 was enacted, it repealed earlier legislation[40] and vested the *parens patriae* power dealing with the 'property and other affairs' of the incompetent in the Court of Protection, allowing for the appointment of a guardian with wide ranging powers. Thus it is argued that the 1959 legislation impliedly removed the court's common law power over incompetent adults. The Mental Health Act 1983 then abolished the power of guardians to consent to medical treatment, but did not reinstate the pre-existing power of the court. The court's protective wardship jurisdiction comes to an end when a child reaches majority.

Thus when faced with a dilemma the court will look at all the factors and make an order as to the lawfulness[41] of any proposed course of action, be it treatment or withdrawal. A declaration of lawfulness is not the same as consent. Valid consent is a complete defence in the event of litigation, but a declaration of lawfulness can be challenged, as indeed it was in Re S.[42]

THE FUTURE

Case law is developing gradually in the area of living wills and appears to support their validity, provided that they meet the relevant criteria. Yet, it would seem that legislation is required to clarify some anomalies.

Some jurisdictions, notably Australia have legislated in this area. The Medical Treatment Act 1988 creates an offence of medical trespass, which is committed by a medical practitioner if he knowingly treats otherwise, than in accordance with, the certified wishes of the patient. As such the Act firmly uphold the patient's right to self-determination.

However, the UK Government has no immediate[43] plans to introduce legislation in this area. The House of Lords Select Committee on Medical Ethics 1994 and rejected calls for legislation on living wills. The Law Commission and the BMA have made some recommendations, and while these may act persuasively on judicial decisions, they are not legally binding.

A survey carried out for the Centre of Medical Law and Ethics, King's College, London in 1992 reached the conclusion that while patients were broadly in favour of living wills having the force of law, doctors were largely opposed to such legislation.[44]

However, in August 2002, the General Medical Council (GMC) issued guidance in a document 'Withholding and Withdrawing Life-prolonging Treatment: Good Practice in Decision Making' in which it states

> Any valid advance refusal of treatment – one made when the patient was competent and on the basis of adequate information about the implications of his/her choice – is legally binding and must be respected where it is clearly applicable to the patient's present circumstances and where there is no reason to believe that the patient had changed his/her mind

It could be argued that this does no more than restate the law as it currently exists. Thus legislation is required for there to be any change to the law.

There are advantages and disadvantages to legislation. One perceived advantage is that if doctors were legally obliged to follow the instructions in a living will, they would be similarly obliged to take a more pro-active role in discussions with the patient about his future in the context of life sustaining treatment. Another advantage would be that a doctor could be granted civil and criminal immunity when withdrawing life sustaining treatment in accordance with the instructions in a living will.

However, one potential disadvantage is that it would remove the flexibility from treatment choices, where the patient had limited or no residual powers of communication and wished to change his mind.

Arguably the most damaging outcome of such legislation would be the development of a climate of distrust between the patient and doctor. The patient may fear that in the face of a legally binding living will, the doctor might act prematurely in withdrawing treatment, rather than waiting until such time as dictated by the patient. Thus it would seem that in the foreseeable future it is unlikely that there will be any significant changes to the legal status of living wills in the UK.

REFERENCES, NOTES AND FURTHER READING

1. Such an event might take the form of persistent vegetative state (PVS); coma; terminal illness or when the patient may be faced with a serious diagnosis and a range of treatment options.

2. *Pretty v United Kingdom (Application 2346/02)*, 2001, 2 FCR 97, in which the impact of the Human Rights Act was considered and it was held that the right to life does not imply a correlative right to die.

3. A number of societies and organisations have produced their own versions, such as The Terrence Higgins Trust, Voluntary Euthanasia Society, The Patients Association, Legal Systems Ltd.

4. *Re R*, 1991, 4 ALL ER 177.

5. *R v Portsmouth Hospital Ex p Glass*, 1999, 50 BMLR 269 (CA).

6. *Re J (A Minor) (Child in Care: Medical Treatment)*, 1993, Fam 15; 1992, 4 ALL ER 614 CA.

7. *Ibid.* at 41.

8. *Re R*, 1991, 4 ALL ER 177 at 184.

9. The principle of autonomy was used as one of the justifications for separating the conjoined twins, Mary and Jody in 2000, *Re A*, 2000, 3 FCR 577.

10. *F v West Berkshire Health Authority*, 1990, 2 AC 1 HL in which Lord Goff referred to 'conduct beyond that which is acceptable in everyday life'.

11. *Schloendorff v Society of New York Hospital*, 105 NE 92, New York, 1914.

12. *Re T (Adult: Refusal of Treatment)*, 1993, CA; *Malette v Shulman*, 1990, 67 DLR (4th) 321.

13. *Re S (Adult: Refusal of Medical Treatment)*, 1992, 9 BMLR 69, where a woman was given damages for undergoing a 'forced caesarean', despite medical opinion that it was in both her and the baby's best interest; *Re C (Adult)*, 1994, 1 WLR 290 where it was accepted that a man who was schizophrenic could validly refuse to have his gangrenous foot amputated; *Re T (Adult: Refusal of Treatment)*, 1993, CA where the refusal by Jehovah's Witness to a blood transfusion was upheld. Lord Donaldson MR said 'The patient's choice exists whether the reasons for making that choice are rational, irrational, unknown or even non-existent.' p 113.

14. Cruzan v Director, Missouri Department of Health (1990) 110 S Ct 2841. In this case the Supre Court considered whether Nancy Cruzan, who had been severely injured in an automobile accident and was in a persistent regetative state, had a right under the United States constitution which would require the hospital to withdraw life-sustaining treatment at her parents' request 1990, 110 S Ct 2841.

15. *Re S (Adult: Refusal of Medical Treatment)*, 1992, 9 BMLR 69.

16. *Malette v Shulman*, 1987; affd (1990) CA.

17. *Airedale NHS Trust v Bland*, 1993, 1 ALL ER 821.

18. Discussed post.

19. *Re W (A Minor: Refusal of Treatment)*, 1992, 4 ALL ER 627 (CA); *Re R (a minor)*, 1993, 2 FLR 757. A 16-year old with anorexia who refused treatment was found not to be competent on the basis that her condition forced her to refuse and a 16-year old with psychotic tendencies who refused medication while lucid, was also not competent to refuse.

20. Sanctity of Life was discussed in Ms B (ante) and *Re A* conjoined twins. *Re J* in which it was said that sometimes sanctity of life must yield to self-determination.
21. *Re MB (An Adult: Medical Treatment)*, 1997, 38 BMLR 175 (CA).
22. *Sidaway v Bethlem Royal Hospital Governors*, 1984, 1 ALL ER 1018 (CA), affd (1985) HL. The patient underwent an operation which carried with it an interest 1%–2% risk of damage to the spinal cord. The patient was not warned of the risk, which did in fact materialise and she became severely disabled. The woman brought an action in tort, arguing that her consent to the operation had not been valid, an the basis that she would not have consented was valid, in that she had been informed of the general nature of the operation. The Court went on to say that a doctor is not negligent if he acts in accordance with a responsible body of medical opinion (the Bolam Test), and that this approach applies to the amount of information the doctor chooses to give to the patient as well as to the type of treatment he recommends. Lord Bridge referred to 'particular risks' and said that the need to disclose such risks, might be so obvious, that no reasonably prudent medical man would fail to inform the patient of it.
23. President's Commission: *Deciding to Forgo Life-Sustaining Treatment* 1983, US.
24. *Airedale NHS Trust v Bland*, 1993, 1 ALL ER 821.
25. *B v A NHS Hospital Trust*, 2002, EWHC 429 (Fam).
26. *Re T (Adult: Refusal of Medical Treatment)*, 1992, 4 ALL ER 649.
27. *Airedale NHS Trust v Bland*, 1993, 1 ALL ER 821.
28. *ibid* at 860.
29. *B v A NHS Hospital Trust*, 2002, EWHC 429 (Fam).
30. *Airedale NHS Trust v Bland*, 1993, 1 ALL ER 821@866.
31. *Re C (Adult: Refusal of Treatment)*, 1994, 1 WLR 290.
32. Law Commission No. 321,1995 para 5.24.
33. *Re AK (Adult Patient) (Medical Treatment: Consent)*, 2001, 1 FLR 129; 2001, 58 BMLR 151.
34. Clews G. 'Doctors back patients' right to refuse treatment', 2002, *BMA News*, 30 March p 12.
35. With some statutory exceptions, such as treatment given under the Mental Health Acts.
36. *T v T*, 1988, Fam 52.
37. *Re T (Adult: Refusal of Medical Treatment)*, 1992, 9 BMLR 46 (CA).
38. *Cruzan v Director*, Missouri Department of Health, 1990, 110 S Ct 2841.
39. *Re F (Mental Patient: Sterilisation)*, 1990, 2 AC 1.
40. Lunacy and Mental Treatment Acts 1890 to 1930, and the Mental Deficiency Acts 1913 to 1938.
41. The Court's jurisdiction derives from RSC Ord 15 r 16.
42. *Re S (Adult: Refusal of Medical Treatment)*, 1992, 9 BMLR 69.
43. The Government has promised a draft Bill on incapacity, which is intended to give carers or close relatives legal authority to make day-to-day welfare and medical as well as financial decisions, but not in this parliamentary session. The Times, 14 Jan 2003.
44. However, it should be noted that this survey was carried out in a climate of uncertainty, engendered by the publicity surrounding HIV/AIDs.

13

Euthanasia and end-of-life decision-making

Hazel Biggs

INTRODUCTION

As medical technology advances and it becomes increasingly possible to keep people alive who previously would have died, medical professionals and the public have been exercised by issues of death and dying. For some the possibility of extended life in a debilitated condition may not be preferable, while the ideals of others who seek perpetual life and youth may not be possible. Inevitably tensions will arise when it comes to making medical decisions about these boundaries. Life and death are traditionally the domain of the medical profession but at a time of rapid legal and medical development medical professionals need to be certain that their practise accords with the law and ethics.

In a climate of enhanced patient autonomy and following a number of high profile legal cases[1] and permissive legal reforms or attitudes in other jurisdictions, repeated public opinion polls suggest that there is significant support for assisted dying.[2] Generally patients wish to be involved in medical decision-making and to retain control of their lives until they die. For some, as Ronald Dworkin explains, this means requesting or seeking assistance to die, 'everyday rational people all over the world plead to be allowed to die. Sometimes they plead for others to kill them. Some of them are dying already.... Some of them want to die because they are unwilling to live in the only way left open to them'.[3] As a result medical practitioners are increasingly likely to be involved in end-of-life decision-making and to encounter patients seeking assisted dying. Treatment withdrawal decisions, treatment refusal, requests for assisted dying through active intervention or assisted suicide, and advance directives are becoming commonplace. These areas will be discussed in order to assess how doctors can and should respond within established legal and ethical codes.

DEFINITIONS

The law responds differently depending on the kind of conduct involved, therefore it is important that the distinctions and definitions are well understood. Dictionary definitions of euthanasia speak of 'mercy killing', which is generally thought to be derived from the Greek ideal of the good death where *eu* means good and *thanatos* means death.[4] Active euthanasia amounts to positive action taken with the intention of ending a person's life. By contrast passive euthanasia results from conduct that results in death but does not apparently involve active intervention aimed at causing death. Thus non-treatment, withdrawal of treatment and double effect are all regarded as examples of passive euthanasia. Passive and active euthanasia may be categorised as voluntary, where the patient requests the intervention and colludes with it, or non-voluntary, which means that the patient is unable to participate in the decision-making process and effectively becomes the object of the end-of-life decision rather than a party to it. Treatment decisions of this type will usually be taken by the carers and medical team. A third category defined by some commentators as involuntary euthanasia refers to euthanasia against the will of the patient or victim. Such conduct is clearly always criminal and should be regarded as homicide rather than as part of medical decision-making.

END-OF-LIFE DECISIONS

End-of-life decision-making can take many forms. The legal approach differs depending on the circumstances and the boundaries between those practices that are considered lawful and those which are not complex. The basic legal position is that active killing is homicide, murder or manslaughter. Even if the patient requests intervention and consents to it 'the law does not leave the issue in the hands of doctors; it treats euthanasia as murder.'[5] However, rapid medical advancement alongside often misleading media reporting of controversial cases introduces uncertainty when applied to the myriad of situations clinicians encounter everyday. Perhaps the most logical way to discuss these is to apply the definitions as above to practical scenarios and decided legal cases. This chapter will use the prominent cases of R v Cox[6] and Pretty v UK,[7] to illustrate many of the complex legal principles involved in euthanasia and end-of-life decision-making where the patient is competent to decide for herself. Alongside these issues the methods of deciding for patients who lack decision-making capacity will be discussed in relation to cases concerning patients in permanent vegetative state (PVS) through the lens of the decision in Airedale NHS Trust v Bland.

ENDING SUFFERING BY ENDING LIFE

Consultant rheumatologist Dr Nigel Cox had been treating Mrs Lillian Boyes for rheumatoid arthritis for a number of years. As her condition deteriorated and she became terminally ill she began to request assistance to die. She suffered unbearable pain, which was not relieved by the treatment Dr Cox provided. The patient and her family felt that there was nothing to be gained by prolonging her agony.

Ultimately Dr Cox elected to inject Mrs Boyes with strong potassium chloride, which has no therapeutic benefit in this context, and Mrs Boyes died shortly afterwards. The family was relieved that her suffering was over and Dr Cox recorded what had happened in the patient's notes. A short time later a ward sister made a report to the police explaining what had occurred and Dr Cox was charged, initially with murder. However, in order to convict a person of murder it must be demonstrated that an action was performed with the intention of causing death and that death did indeed result.[8] In this case, because Mrs Boyes had been cremated before the police investigation began, it was not possible to establish the precise cause of death.[9] Dr Cox had performed the positive action of injecting Mrs Boyes with a lethal substance expecting that she would die, and shortly afterwards she did die, but she was also terminally ill and there was always the chance, however remote, that death resulted from natural causes. It could be inferred from his conduct[10] in administering a drug known to cause death and having no therapeutic value in this context, that he intended her death. But it could not be established that he had, in fact, caused her death. So Dr Cox was charged with attempted murder and convicted.

As is usual when a medical practitioner is convicted of such a serious crime, the doctor's case was subsequently heard by the General Medical Council (GMC). However, like the court, which sentenced him to one year imprisonment, suspended for one year, the GMC was lenient. Very unusually the GMC declined to strike Dr Cox off the medical register, preferring instead to permit him to continue to practise, albeit under supervision for a period and conditional on his undergoing training on pain relief. The level of support for Dr Cox from Mrs Boyes family was persuasive in the GMC hearing, as had been the feelings of the jury in the court case where it was reported that several members wept as the verdict was delivered. The tensions are obvious however.

Mrs Boyes was apparently exercising her autonomy, with the support of her family, in repeatedly requesting that her doctor help her to die. The law states that 'every patient of sound mind and adult years has the right to decide what shall be done with his body'[11] which means that patients have an absolute right to refuse treatment 'even if a refusal may risk personal injury or even lead to premature death'[12] as was seen in the recent case of Ms B.[13,14] The right to refuse does not however extend to demanding particular treatments. Furthermore, one must question whether a patient in Mrs Boyes position would have the mental capacity to make such a decision? English law presumes that adult patients do have decision-making capacity, but that is a rebuttable presumption. Capacity is assessed according to whether the patient can comprehend and retain information relevant to the decision to be made and weigh that information in the balance in order to arrive at a decision.[15] While it is not appropriate to suggest that a patient lacks capacity simply because she is terminally ill and in pain it would seem reasonable to suggest that some enquiry should have been made to ascertain whether her capacity was impaired. Every jurisdiction that permits voluntary euthanasia,[16] either as active euthanasia or assisted suicide, incorporates an assessment of capacity and insists that alternative treatments have been considered and that requests should be repeated and in writing, before the patient is allowed to die. Mrs Boyes apparently sought to die, but perhaps she would not have, if adequate symptomatic control had been available.

DOUBLE EFFECT AND LEGAL INTENTION

Dr Cox might have followed a different clinical path. Instead of administering a lethal dose of medication he could have given incrementally increasing doses of recognised pain relieving drugs, an established regimen in terminal care. The legal outcome would have been very different since if this course of action led to the death of the patient Nigel Cox would almost certainly not have been convicted of any criminal wrong doing.

Based on the doctrine of *double effect* this approach was first discussed in this context in the authoritative case of Dr Bodkin Adams.[17] Here it was established that a doctor may '. . . do all that is proper and necessary to relieve pain and suffering, even if the measures he takes may incidentally shorten life'.[18] The problem for Cox was that the action he took was not regarded as 'proper and necessary' and the measures he employed could be expected to kill his patient rather than 'incidentally' shortening her life. The law distinguishes between Nigel Cox's conduct and the doctrine of *double effect* on the basis of criminal intention. *Double effect* dictates that a good act, i.e. giving a medicine to treat the patient's symptoms, is permissible even if it has 'bad' side effects. The doctor's intention then will be to treat the patient, not to cause her death. Where medication is given that has no therapeutic benefit the doctors intention can only be to cause the patient's death, hence it is not lawful.

TREATMENT WITHDRAWAL

The legal position in relation to patients in persistent vegetative state (PVS) who are unable to participate in the decision-making process is rather different. Such patients are not terminally ill and can be kept alive almost indefinitely. They will require intensive support for their lives to be sustained and the only benefit to be gained is that life is prolonged. The quality of that life is however questionable as these patients can never recover from their condition and no treatment will improve their prognosis. Arguably treatment is futile, but can treatment lawfully be withdrawn so that life can come to an end?

A series of cases, commencing with Bland[19] have confirmed that treatment may legitimately be withdrawn in these circumstances. The law does not regard treatment withdrawal as euthanasia because no positive action is being taken to end the patient's life.[20] Instead, if liability were to accrue it would do so as a result of a failure to act, an omission. The law attaches liability to failures to act only where there is a legal duty to act, so the limits of the doctor's legal duty to treat is central in cases such as this. Here the duty every doctor to her patients is clear in as much as the patient must be treated according to their best interests. But how are 'best interests' to be defined? Recent cases suggest that best interests do not encompass only medical best interests but that the social and welfare implications of any treatment decision should also be considered[21] suggesting that a broad definition be adopted.

The Law Commission has reviewed best interests criteria on a number of occasions[22] and recommended *inter alia* that the ascertainable past and present wishes of the person be considered[23] along with the views of relevant others (though these should not be definitive), the factors that the person themselves might consider were they able, and the characteristics of the treatment under consideration, particularly whether or not there is a less invasive or restrictive alternative. Although no legislation has yet been implemented it seems likely that a system of proxy decision-making, similar to that permissible under the Adults with Incapacity (Scotland) Act 2000 will be adopted in the near future.[24] Other jurisdictions[25] already legislate for proxy decision-making or operate systems of substituted judgement and it is hoped that such legislation will plug the legal lacuna in England that currently means that nobody has authority to consent to treatment on behalf of an adult patient who lacks capacity. Similarly there have been calls for the law on assisted suicide to be liberalised in line with some other jurisdictions.

ASSISTED SUICIDE

Assisted suicide occurs when a person enlists the help of another in order to end her own life. Legally it is distinguished from active euthanasia and homicide because it is the patient rather than the 'assistant' who performs the final act that results in death. Generally assisted suicide will occur where a person is physically unable to complete the act of suicide due to physical impairment that restricts access to the means of committing suicide.[26] In Holland, assisted suicide is regarded as euthanasia and is permissible under the patient assisted dying legislation, which allows medically assisted dying where procedural guidelines are closely adhered to.[27] In Oregon assisted suicide has been legal since 1998.[28] In both jurisdictions safeguards have been introduced to ensure that assistance is provided only after repeated requests over a stipulated period of time, by appropriately qualified medical personnel and that patients are properly diagnosed and have received all available medical care. However in England, assisted suicide is prohibited and carries a maximum penalty of 14 years imprisonment under Section 2 of the Suicide Act 1961. Section 1 of the Act decrees that suicide itself is no longer a crime but there is no *right* to suicide.

The recent case brought by Diane Pretty challenged the law on assisted suicide through the domestic courts at every level and ultimately in the European Court of Human Rights.[29] Diane Pretty was diagnosed with motor neurone disease at the age of forty and when she discovered the details of the likely manner of her death she decided that she would want to die before her condition reached its inevitable conclusion. She also knew however that by that stage she would be unable to kill herself and would need help. Initially she sought assistance from her doctors but none were prepared to break the law to assist her. In the alternative her husband was prepared to help but she was unprepared to subject him to criminal prosecution. She asked for an assurance from the Director of Public Prosecutions (DPP) that were her husband to give the help offered he would not be prosecuted. The DPP declined to give such an assurance. There is discretion under the Suicide Act 1961[30] for the DPP to decide whether or not to prosecute but the courts held that the discretion could only be exercised after the event.[31]

Her second claim was that UK law discriminated against her because she was unable to commit suicide herself due to her physical impairment and the state was preventing her from obtaining assistance to do what an able-bodied person could achieve alone. Her claim was brought under Articles 2, 3, 8, 9 and 14 of the European Convention of Human Rights. She argued that under Article 2 the right to life included a right to die at a time and in a manner of her choosing, which the courts failed to recognise. Her Article 3 claim against being subjected to inhuman and degrading treatment failed because it was her disease rather than the state that was causing her suffering. Only Article 8, respect for private life, was viewed sympathetically on the understanding that person's autonomy and the ability to exercise it is becoming a central part of life. Article 9 refers to freedom of thought, consciousness and religion and was summarily dismissed as Mrs Pretty's views did not manifest a religious belief. Article 14 articulated the discrimination claim and was dismissed on the basis that it was her medical condition that prevented her from committing suicide, not the state. The law applied equally to all and anyway there is no *right* to suicide to be protected. The claim was ultimately rejected however, because the state has a duty to protect the interests of the vulnerable as it decides necessary in spite of the fact that Mrs Pretty's individual rights, as a person who was not vulnerable to the kinds of abuses envisaged in the Suicide Act, were effectively being subverted to the potential rights of nameless individuals.

Diane Pretty's case is not an isolated one. In 1993 Sue Rodriguez, who also suffered from Motor Neurone Disease, brought a constitutional challenge against the Canadian Criminal Code,[32] alleging that she was being discriminated against. Her case was defeated by the narrowest of margins with many of the judges expressing sympathy with her plight. Similar cases have been heard in the USA[33] but the outcome has always been the same.

Yet assisted dying, and assisted suicide in particular remains a topical issue. Recent months have witnessed a succession of people travelling from England to Switzerland to avail themselves of the services of Dignitas, an organisation that will arrange for assisted suicide. In Switzerland assisted suicide is not a crime if it is done for compassionate motives but it is currently unregulated. These death tourists can make the necessary arrangements in advance and be assisted to die within hours of arriving in Switzerland. There is no requirement that the person is terminally ill or suffering unbearably, as there is in Holland and Oregon, and they may not even be examined by a doctor prior to the suicidal act.

CONCLUSIONS

It seems clear from the public debate of Diane Pretty's case, opinion polls and the recent incidents of death tourism that the demand for assisted dying will continue to increase and with it calls for permissive legal reform. Alongside this there are obvious tensions between the legal approach to mentally incapacitated patients who cannot speak for themselves and the legal response to those who make competent demands for assistance in dying. Similarly concerns are being voiced about the apparent inhumanity of permitting incapacitated adults to die slowly through withdrawal of nutrition and hydration.[34] How much longer can the law reconcile a position on allowing decisions to be made that effectively allow those who cannot decide for themselves to die in a slow and potentially distressing manner while others who wish to die quickly and painlessly are prevented from so doing? Legal reform is overdue.

REFERENCES AND NOTES

1. *Airedale NHS Trust v Bland*, 1993, 1 All ER 821, R (on the application of Pretty) v DPP 2001, All ER 1, Re B (Adult: Refusal of Medical Treatment), 2002, 2 Au El 449.
2. Four National Opinion Polls conducted for the Voluntary Euthanasia Society between 1976 and 1993 indicate support for euthanasia where a person is suffering from an intolerable incurable physical illness and has requested such help rising from 69% to 79%.
3. Dworkin R, *Life's Dominion: An Argument about Abortion and Euthanasia,* London: Harper Collins, 1993, p 179.
4. It is interesting to note that in Greece euthanasia is not permitted and clinicians tend to practise rather more conservatively than those in many other countries, avoiding practices like double effect and terminal sedation that have become routine in other jurisdictions.
5. Williams G, *Textbook of Criminal Law*, 2nd edn, London: Stevens, 1983, p 580.
6. *R v Cox*, 1992, 12 BMLR 38.
7. *R (on the application of Pretty) v DPP*, 2001, EWHC Admin 788; 2002, 1 All ER 1.
8. *R v White*, 1910, 2 KB 124.
9. Arguably, because of the method used in this case, it would always have been difficult to establish, beyond a reasonable doubt, that death was caused by the potassium chloride injection.

10. *R v Nedrick*, 1986, 3 All ER 1.
11. *Schloendorf v Society of New York Hospital*, 1914 105 NE 92, per Cardozo J.
12. *Re T (An Adult) (Consent to medical treatment)*, 1992, 4 All ER 649.
13. *Re B (Adult: Refusal of Medical Treatment)*, 2002, 2 All ER 449.
14. Ms B was not terminally ill but was permanently disabled and dependent upon mechanical life support. She chose not to continue living in that way and refused further treatment, insisting that the mechanical life support be withdrawn. The court upheld her claim and she died soon after.
15. *Re MB (An Adult: Medical treatment)*, 1997, 2 FCR 541, 8 Med LR 217.
16. The Netherlands and Oregon both insist on these measures, as did the Australian Northern Territory legislation before it was repealed. The Patient Assisted Dying Bill (2003), which was presented as a Private Members bill in the House of Lords, included similar safeguards.
17. *R v Adams*, The Times, 9th April 1957.
18. H. Palmer, 'Dr Adams' Trial for Murder', 1957, *Crim. LR* 365, at 375.
19. *Airedale NHS Trust v Bland*, 1993, 1 All ER 821.
20. Despite the courts insistence that withdrawal of treatment is not euthanasia it is clear that conduct such as this does fall within the definition of passive euthanasia since it has the death of the patient as its aim.
21. *Re SL (Adult Patient: Medical Treatment)*, 2000, 2 FCR 452.
22. Law Commission Consultation Paper 129, *Mentally Incapacitated Patients and Decision making*, London: HMSO, 1993; Law Commission Report 231, *Mental Incapacity*, London: HMSO, 1995.
23. Advance directives would be beneficial here.
24. The government has recently undertaken a public consultation on these issues and seems virtually certain to introduce legislation to this effect in the near future.
25. Most notably many of states in America.
26. For example where a person is immobilised and therefore prevented from obtaining access to medication and needs it to be brought to them.
27. For a thorough discussion of euthanasia in the Netherlands see, De Haan J, 'The New Dutch Law on Euthanasia', 2002, *Med LR*, 10: 57–75.
28. Death with Dignity Act, 1998.
29. *R (On the Application of Pretty) v DPP*, 2001, EWHC Admin 788; 2002, 1 All ER 1, *Pretty v United Kingdom*, 2002, 2 F.C.R. 97.
30. S2(4).
31. See Tur R. 'Legislative Technique and Human rights: the Sad Case of Assisted Suicide' *Crim. LR*, 2003, 3–12, for an interesting argument suggesting that this point was misconstrued by the courts.
32. *Rodriguez v A-G of British Columbia*, 1993, 3 WWR 553.
33. *State of Washington et al. v Glucksberg et al.*, 1997, S Ct 2258, and *Vacco et al. v Quill*, 1997, 117 S Ct 2293.
34. Craig GM, 'On Withholding Nutrition and Hydration in the Terminally Ill: has Palliative Medicine Gone too far?' *J. Med. Ethics*, 1994, 139–143, Biggs H, *Euthanasia, Death with Dignity and the Law*. Oxford: Hart, 2001.

14

Abortion and reproductive health

Adrian Lower

INTRODUCTION

The field of human reproduction continues to challenge both the medicolegal and ethical boundaries of common experience. In this chapter the issues relating to abortion and contraception will be summarised and the legal framework under which rulings have been made in relation to fertility treatments will be discussed.

ABORTION

It is a criminal offence contrary to the Offences against the Person Act 1861 and the Abortion Act 1967 (as amended) for any person ' ... with intent to procure the miscarriage of any woman, whether she be or be not with child ...' unless this is carried out under the specific conditions laid down by the Abortion Act.

There has been substantial legal debate over the definition of 'miscarriage'. Some authorities[1] hold the view that as soon as the ovum is fertilised it is 'carried' in the woman's body. This would effectively make postcoital contraception illegal unless carried out in accordance with the Abortion Act. Others[2,3] take the view that it is only truly carried and thus capable of miscarriage from the time of implantation. In practice the Attorney General's statement[4] in 1983 which favoured the implantation argument means that no prosecution will result from postcoital contraception. Indeed post coital contraceptives are now available as over the counter medicines from pharmacies in the UK.

The common law of homicide can only apply once a baby has been born. Therefore, in order to protect the life of a child *in utero* but considered 'capable of being born alive' the Infant Life (Preservation) Act was introduced in 1929 embodying the offence of child destruction. In 1967 at the time of the original Abortion Act a gestational age of 28 weeks was considered to be the earliest stage at which a child could be capable of being born alive. Advances in neonatal intensive care have moved that milestone a little earlier to 24 weeks of gestation. The amendment of the Abortion Act by the Human Fertilisation and Embryology Act 1990 changed from 28 weeks to 24 weeks the gestational age at which a routine termination could legally be carried out. The grounds for termination are summarised in Table 14.1.

Selective termination in which one or more fetuses forming part of a multiple pregnancy are selectively aborted has been given recognition under the amendments to the Act, provided it is undertaken for one of the grounds above.

Some health professionals have religious or ethical objections to abortion and the original Abortion Act 1967 contains a clause allowing non-participation on grounds of conscience. How far does non-participation extend? In 1987 Mrs Janaway, a medical secretary sought judicial review to overturn her employer's decision to terminate her contract because she had refused to type a letter of referral for abortion on grounds of conscience. Her application was refused and in 1988 the House of Lords dismissed her appeal.[5] It was held that 'participation' meant 'taking part in treatment' and not merely arrangements preliminary to treatment.

There have been differences of opinion between the prospective parents as to whether a pregnancy should be terminated. The case of Paton v Trustees of BPAS and another [1978][6] and C and another v S and another [1987][7] established that a father had no authority to

---

Table 14.1 Grounds for termination of a pregnancy.

Abortion Act 1967 (as amended by Section 37 of the Human Fertilisation and Embryology Act 1990)

a that the pregnancy has not exceeded its 24th week and that continuation of the pregnancy would involve risk, greater than if the pregnancy were terminated, of injury to the physical or mental health of the pregnant woman or any existing children of her family; or

b that the termination is necessary to prevent grave permanent injury to the physical or mental health of the pregnant woman; or

c that the continuance of the pregnancy would involve risk to the life of the pregnant woman, greater than if the pregnancy were terminated; or

d that there is a substantial risk that if the child were born it would suffer from such physical or mental abnormalities as to be seriously handicapped.

prevent the mother undergoing a termination nor could the fetus *in utero* be a party to an action whilst it was unborn.

CONTRACEPTION

Contraception has never been banned in the UK as it has in some countries. Medicolegal difficulties arise in two areas and relate primarily to issues of consent: the young person and the handicapped person.

THE YOUNG PERSON

Currently up to 26% of girls report having had sexual intercourse under the age of 16, therefore appropriate contraceptive advice is important to reduce the incidence of teenage pregnancy in England and Wales. A Department of Health and Social Security (DHSS) circular published in 1974 and revised in 1980 advised that if a girl under the age of 16 did not wish her parents to be told of her request for contraception then those wishes should be respected although every effort should be made to encourage parental involvement in her decision. This advice was challenged by Mrs Gillick a mother of 4 daughters who sought assurance from her local health authority that no advice regarding contraception or abortion would be given to her daughters without her prior knowledge and agreement. When this reassurance was not forthcoming, Mrs Gillick sought a court declaration that the DHSS advice was unlawful and wrong. The case eventually reached the House of Lords in 1985 who upheld the DHSS advice by a margin of three to two. The Gillick judgment may be summarised thus: a doctor would be justified in providing contraceptive advice to a girl under the age of 16 provided he was satisfied she could understand his advice; he could not persuade her to involve her parents; she was likely to have sexual intercourse and that, unless contraceptive advice was given, her physical and/or mental health was likely to suffer[8]. Further legislation, particularly the Children Act 1989 with its concept of parental responsibility rather than parental right, has further reinforced that concept.

THE MENTALLY HANDICAPPED PATIENT

Control of fertility in a mentally handicapped patient is a common problem faced by medical practitioners. The legal position regarding sterilisation has been clarified by the House of Lords decision in the case of F v West Berkshire Health Authority.[9] It was held that an adult woman incapable of giving informed consent because of mental impairment could be sterilised, provided the operation was considered to be in her best interests. This is defined as treatment carried out to 'either save the patient's life or ensure improvement or prevent deterioration in the patient's physical or mental health'. What constitutes best practice is a matter to be decided by the doctor in accordance with good professional practice as defined by a reasonable body of medical opinion. In practice an application should be made to the court for a declaration that the proposed procedure is lawful in an individual case. The steps to be followed are set out in the Department of Health's Circular HC(90)22 revised in 1992. Where sterilisation is not the primary aim of the treatment, as in the case of hysterectomy for intractable menorrhagia, Court approval need not be obtained,[10] provided other less radical treatments are not appropriate and the recommendation is supported by two consultant colleagues. Termination of pregnancy also requires no preliminary Court approval provided it is performed in accordance with the Abortion Act and in the best interests of the patient.[11] No powers exist under the Mental Health Act 1983 to sanction such a procedure when the patient herself is incapable of giving informed consent[12] neither can a relative give consent on the patient's behalf.

The clinician's opinion should be carefully documented in the medical records and where there is any doubt medicolegal advice should be sought.

INFERTILITY

It is in the treatment of infertility that perhaps the most challenging ethical and medicolegal dilemmas occur. The Human Fertilisation and Embryology Act 1990 established legislation for the protection of patients undergoing fertility treatment and the 'as yet' unborn child under the auspices of the Human Fertilisation and Embryology Authority (HFEA). The HFEA was the first statutory body of its kind in the world. The primary objective is the licensing and monitoring of clinics and centres carrying out *in vitro* fertilisation, donor insemination and human embryo research. (This includes regulation of the storage of gametes and embryos.) This remit to licence embryo research was expanded to incorporate new regulations passed in January 2001 enabling the use of embryos for research into causes and treatment of serious disease.

One of the central themes of the HFEA is the issue of confidentiality. Initially confidentiality was so tight that doctors in a licensed fertility clinic could not even write to the referring doctor with details of treatment undergone nor use information from their notes to defend themselves in the event of a medicolegal problem arising. This has now been relaxed by the Human Fertilisation and Embryology (Disclosure of Information) Act 1992.

The HFEA produces a Code of Practice providing guidance to clinics in interpreting the statutes of the Act. All licensed clinics must adhere to this code of practice and undergo annual inspection and audit to confirm that they do so. In addition to licensing and inspecting clinics the HFEA is also required to keep a register of information about donors, treatments and children born as a result of treatment and provide advice, information and support to patients, donors and clinics. The register will allow any young person of 16 years of age or older who is due to marry to enquire whether they were born as a result of egg or sperm donation and if so, whether they are genetically related to their intended husband or wife. Any one of 18 years of age will also be able to enquire whether they are the product of donated sperm or eggs whether or not they intend to marry.

Currently all sperm donors and egg donors are protected from having any identifying information about them released to their genetic offspring. There is pressure however that this anonymity be withdrawn as it is not perceived to be in the best interests of the child to be denied identifying information about his or her genetic parent. Not only is there pressure to change the law for the future, but some authorities are keen to see this reversed retrospectively. Many fertility specialists fear that such legislation will put off potential donors and lead to a shortage of donor gametes. Retrospective changes in the legislation will also impact on the rights of the donors who provided their gametes in the belief that they would enjoy anonymity. These changes in legislation are currently the subject of wide public consultation.

The HFEA also has a statutory responsibility to review research developments that relate to human embryology, and to advise the Secretary of State in England and Wales and others on the relevance of this research to existing and new clinical practice and policy.

There have been a number of high profile cases in which laboratory procedures have allowed errors of identification of gametes to occur resulting in the distressing situation where a couple have found out after the birth of their child or children that they are not the genetic parents. This issue was handled with great sensitivity by Dame Elizabeth Butler-Sloss, President of the Family Division.[13] Subsequently the HFEA has issued guidance to clinics such that robust witnessing procedures are in place each time an opportunity arises in the lab for mixing gametes or embryos. Such a policy should substantially reduce the chance of similar errors occurring in the future.

Multiple pregnancy is one of the major complications of assisted conception with implications for the health of both mother and fetuses. Initially a maximum of three embryos could be replaced but as *in vitro* fertilisation (IVF) procedures have become more successful, the HFEA has directed that only in exceptional cases should three embryos be replaced and it is hoped this will lead to a reduction in multiple births and the associated problems of prematurity.

The other major issue which has led to distress and misunderstanding is that of storage of gametes and embryos and the conditions surrounding their disposal. Gametes and embryos are permitted to be stored initially for a period of 5 years. This period may be extended in certain circumstances laid down under the The Human Fertilisation and Embryology (Statutory Storage Period for Embryos) Regulations 1996. Essentially these regulations state that provided specific permission is given by the genetic mother and father of the embryos or gametes and certain other conditions satisfied those embryos may be stored for a further period of five years. If for any reason the clinic is unable to contact the individuals concerned to extend the storage period, then the default position is that the embryos or gametes must be destroyed in accordance with the Human Fertilisation and Embryology Act 1990. The only exception to this is men undergoing vasectomy.

Section 14(3) of the Human Fertilisation and Embryology Act 1990 states that the statutory storage period in respect of gametes is 10 years. Regulations made by Parliament in 1991 allowed for an extension to this storage period in certain circumstances. The Regulations allow for the extension of the statutory storage period if the gametes were provided by a person:

  i whose fertility since providing them has, or is likely to become, in the written opinion of a medical practitioner, significantly impaired;
 ii who was aged under 45 on the date on which the gametes were provided; and
iii who intends the gametes for his own use only.

The HFEA have agreed that men who satisfy ii) and iii) above and who have stored sperm prior to a vasectomy do fulfil the criteria set out in the Regulations and are, therefore, eligible for extended storage.

SURROGACY

Surrogacy arrangements are currently legal in the UK provided that no fee is either demanded or paid. There are two forms of surrogacy arrangement each with its own potential hazards – full surrogacy and host or IVF surrogacy. In full surrogacy the surrogate mother is usually inseminated with the sperm of the commissioning man either within a licensed fertility clinic in which case the Human Fertilisation and Embryology Act applies and the commissioning man is treated as a known sperm donor so that the sperm must be quarantined for 6 months before insemination takes place; or as a private arrangement by vaginal insemination of semen from the commissioning man into the surrogate. This latter arrangement exposes the surrogate to potential infection and is much less likely to be successful than intrauterine insemination of washed, prepared frozen-thawed sperm in a fertility clinic. In host surrogacy the eggs and sperm from the commissioning couple are used to create an embryo that is not genetically related to the surrogate mother which is then implanted in her uterus by a standard embryo transfer technique. Frozen-thawed embryos are usually used for this purpose again to minimise the risk of infection but interestingly this is not mandatory. In practice the legal and counselling process is likely to take considerably longer than 6 months so cryopreservation of embryos prior to a surrogacy arrangement is the norm.

The law recognises the birth mother as the legal parent of the child and commissioning parents must obtain a parental order under Section 30 of the Human Fertilisation and Embryology Act in order to become recognised as the legal parents of the child. The key provisions of Section 30 provide that:

i   The commissioning couple applying for a parental order must be over 18, married and at least one of them must be domiciled in the UK or the Channel Islands or the Isle of Man.

ii At least one of the couple must be genetically related to the child and the pregnancy must have been established either by IVF or Gamete Intra Fallopian Transfer (GIFT) or by artificial insemination, and not by natural intercourse.

iii The child must already be living with the couple and consent obtained from the surrogate and the child's legal father. The surrogacy arrangement must have been implemented.

iv Most importantly the court must be satisfied that 'no money or other benefit (other than for expenses reasonably incurred)' has been paid to the surrogate, *unless authorised by the court.*

If these provisions are not satisfied then the commissioning parents must apply to adopt the child or children. Many couples enter into legal agreements with their surrogate in an attempt to minimise the risk that the surrogate will not give up the child after birth. In fact the 1985 Surrogacy Act makes these agreements practically unenforceable. The risk of a surrogate having a change of heart and not wishing to give up the baby appears to be much lower in host surrogacy cases where the woman is not genetically related to the child.

SEX SELECTION

Sex selection is permitted in the UK in licensed fertility centres under the Human Fertilisation Act 1990 only for the avoidance of sex-linked disorders. Sex selection can be performed at three stages: (i) before conception, where sperm are sorted to produce male and female embryos; (ii) before the embryo is transferred to a woman, where embryos created by IVF are tested to select those of a particular sex for transfer; and (iii) after a pregnancy is established, where termination of pregnancy is used to halt the development of a fetus that is of the unintended sex.

Preconception sex selection is prohibited in licensed clinics except for the prevention of sex linked disorders, but may be carried out in unlicensed centres. The techniques which have been based on various gradient methods or flow cytometry have until recently been unreliable and with uncertain long term effects for the children conceived. Recent work in the US suggests that the results are improving and longer term follow-up will assess any health implications.

Preimplantation genetic diagnosis where embryos created by IVF are 'sexed' usually using Fluorescent *in situ* hybridisation (FISH) is practised in a number of licensed centres in the UK and is the most acceptable and reliable method of sex selection available. A single cell is separated from the developing embryo at around the 8-cell stage and the X and Y chromosomes are labelled using fluorescent markers.

Postimplantation termination of established pregnancies of the 'wrong' sex can legally be terminated under the 1987 Abortion Act provided the risk to the health of the embryo can be demonstrated.

REFERENCES

1. Keown J. Miscarriage: a medicolegal analysis. *Crim. Law Rev.*, 1984, 604–614.
2. Williams G. *Textbook on Criminal Law*, 2nd edn, 294–295. London: Stevens, 1983.

3. Mason JK. *Human Life and Medical Practice*, 90–92. Edinburgh: Edinburgh University Press, 1988.
4. House of Commons: Written Answers, cols 236–237. London: Hansard, May 1983.
5. *Janaway v Salford Health Authority*, 1988, 3 All ER: 1079–1084.
6. *Paton v trustees of BPAS and another*, 1978, 2 All ER: 987–992.
7. *C and another vs and Another*, 1987, 1 All ER: 1230–1244.
8. *Gillick v West Norfolkand Wisbech Area Health Authority and Another*, 1985, 3 All ER: 402–437.
9. *F v West Berkshire Health Authority and Another* (Mental Health Commission intervening), 1989, 2 All ER: 545–571.
10. *Re E (A Minor) (Medical Treatment)*, 7 BMLR:117–119. London: Butterworths, 1991.
11. *Re G The Times*: January 1991.
12. *T v T and Another*, 1988, 1 All ER: 613–625.
13. *Leeds Teaching Hospitals NHS Trust v A and Others*, 2003, EWHC 259.

15

The Children Act 1989*

Allan Levy Q.C.

The Children Act 1989 is landmark legislation by any standards. Even allowing for political hyperbole, there is some force in the observation of one minister, when introducing the bill in parliament, that it is the most comprehensive and far-reaching reform of child law in living memory. The Act has over a hundred sections and 15 schedules and over 30 sets of Rules and Regulations. The long title of the statute gives an indication of its comprehensive nature: 'An Act to reform the law relating to children; to provide for local authority services for children in need and others; to amend the law with respect to children's homes, community homes, voluntary homes and voluntary organisations; to make provision with respect to fostering, child minding and day care for young children, and adoption; and for connected purposes'. The legislation was passed in 1989 but not implemented until October 1991.[1]

Background

In the early 1980's it became abundantly clear that reform of the law regarding children was a priority. Parts of it were ultimately and accurately described in Parliament as 'confusing, piecemeal, outdated, often unfair and in important respects ineffective .... Most notably when it comes to our ability to protect children at risk'. In 1982 the House of Commons Social Services Select Committee began consideration of the issue, and concluded in 1984 that a review of child law was overdue.

Later in 1987 the Cleveland affair, which led to a public inquiry and the influential Cleveland Report,[2] burst on an unsuspecting Britain. This alerted the public to the problems of diagnosing child sexual abuse and the real dangers of overreaction to suspected abuse. The allegations

---

* © Allan Levy Q.C. (2003)

were to a significant extent based upon a controversial medical test relating to physical signs of sexual abuse: reflex anal dilatation. There were considerable delays in the cases coming to court and there was great concern about the medical, social work and legal procedures and practices adopted. The comprehensive report produced after a judicial inquiry[3] acted as a substantial trigger to reform of the law.

A succession of inquiries[4] into the deaths of children resulting from child abuse further fuelled the impetus to reform. Critical comments from the European Court of Human Rights in Strasbourg in a number of cases concerning child care issues[5] also helped. In addition the decision of the House of Lords in the case of Gillick[6] was a considerable influence. Central to the case was the question whether a girl under 16 had the legal capacity to consent to a medical examination and treatment. The law lords held that she had the capacity, including the capacity to consent to contraceptive treatment, if she had sufficient maturity and intelligence to understand the nature and implications of the proposed treatment. This decision, essentially about children's rights regarding decision-making, had a major effect on the debate about law reform.

Parallel with the review of child care law, the Law Commission had carried out its own review of child law in respect of the 'private' law of custody, access, guardianship and wardship. It produced a number of working papers and a final Report.[7] The draft Bill which the Law Commission annexed to its Report covered the reviews of both child care law and 'private' child law. This helpfully led to all the public and private law being gathered together in one place, the Children Act 1989, enabling common principles and remedies to be formulated, where possible, regarding both private and public law.

MAIN POLICIES OF THE ACT

Welfare

Section 1(1) of the Act provides that when a court determines any question with respect to the upbringing of a child, the child's welfare shall be the paramount consideration. The limiting words are important and it is not correct to say that the Children Act 1989 always puts the welfare of the child as the paramount consideration. Certain provisions within the Act apply different tests. A court being asked by a local authority to consider, for example, making a care or supervision order under Section 31 (see below) must first decide if the precise threshold condition as to significant harm is proved and the welfare principle is not to be applied at this stage. If the condition is proved then the welfare principle comes into play and Section 1(3) provides a checklist of matters to be taken into account. These include the ascertainable wishes and feelings of the child concerned (considered in the light of his age and understanding) his physical, emotional and educational needs, and the range of powers available to the court under the Act in the proceedings in question.

When the Human Rights Act 1998, which incorporates into domestic law the European Convention on Human Rights, came into force in October 2000 it was thought by some commentators that the welfare principle might be diluted by the Convention's emphasis on the rights of others as well as those of the child. However, that does not appear to be the effect and in the recent case of Youssef v The Netherlands[8] the European Court of Human rights stated that

> In judicial decisions where the rights under Article 8[9] of parents and those of a child are at stake, the child's rights must be the paramount consideration. If any balancing of interests is necessary, the interests of the child must prevail.

Family care

It is fundamental to the legislation that whenever possible children should be brought up and cared for by their own families. The Act's philosophy is that the child in need can be helped most effectively if the local authority, working in partnership with the parents, provides a range and level of services appropriate to the child's needs. Complementary to this approach is the belief that the state, in the form of the local authority, should not be permitted to control a child's life in any way unless strict statutory criteria are met and a court order obtained. Any possible administrative route into care such as a parental rights resolution has been abolished.

Parental responsibility

The Act introduced the concept of parental responsibility. This is defined in Section 3(1) as

> any of the rights, duties, powers, responsibilities and authority which by law a parent of a child has in relation to the child and his property

Although the definition refers to rights, the intention of the legislation is to emphasise the child as a person and not a possession. The impact of the

Human Rights Act 1998 does not alter the position. Powers and duties given to parents exist in order that they can carry out their responsibilities.

No order

The Law Commission considered that orders were sometimes unnecessary and might discourage parties from negotiating arrangements and agreements. In addition an order might deter a parent from remaining involved with a child after separation or divorce. Accordingly, Section 1(5) provides that the court must not make an order unless it considers that to do so would be better for the child than making no order at all.

Delay

The court must have regard to the general principle that delay in determining a question with respect to the upbringing of a child is likely to prejudice the child's welfare.[10] This attempts to meet one of the main criticisms of proceedings relating to children. Rules of Court and a Protocol deal with the particular timetables to be followed.[11]

Contact

When children are removed from home under a court order by a local authority contact with the parents should be maintained, except where it would be dangerous or otherwise harmful to the child. Section 34 of the Act deals in detail with parental contact with children in care.

Services for children in need

A local authority has statutory duties to provide services for children in need. Schedule 2 of the Act sets out an extensive list of services for families and in respect of children looked after by local authorities. Headings in the Schedule include 'Prevention of neglect and abuse', 'Provision of accommodation in order to protect children' and 'Provision for children living with their families'.

Court structures

The Act provides an integrated and improved court structure with all the courts in essence having the same remedies and powers. This principle was important if the previously unsatisfactory practise of forum-shopping (i.e. having in certain circumstances a number of different jurisdictions to choose from and litigate in) was to be ended.

Aims of the Act

The aims of the Act, therefore, are to simplify, to reform, to co-ordinate, to integrate and to make the courts more user-friendly. Just over 10 years after implementation, the Act can be seen to have successfully streamlined child law within a framework that tries to balance the often-competing interests of the child, the parents and the state, and to provide practical and effective measures.

MAIN PROVISIONS OF THE ACT

Some of the more important aspects of public and private law are dealt with briefly in the space available.

Public law

Part IV of the Act (Sections 31–42) deals with the heart of the public law provisions concerning care and supervision. Section 31(2) sets out the threshold conditions, one of which must be proved by the local authority before the court is in a position to consider whether a care or supervision order should be made. A court may only make an order if it is satisfied:

a. that the child concerned is suffering, or is likely to suffer, significant harm; and
b. that harm, or likelihood of harm, is attributable to
   i. the care given to the child, or likely to be given to him if the order were not made, not being what would be reasonable to expect a parent to give to him; or
   ii. the child's being beyond parental control.

Section 31(9) contains important definitions. 'Harm' means ill treatment or the impairment of health or development. Section 120 of the Adoption and Children Act 2002[12] adds to the definition of 'harm' the words, 'including, for example, impairment suffered from seeing or hearing the ill treatment of another'. 'Development' means physical, intellectual, emotional, social or behavioural development. 'Health' means physical or mental health; and 'ill-treatment' includes sexual abuse and forms of ill treatment which are not physical. 'Significant' is not defined and appears, as a result of lack of reported cases, not to have caused any difficulty in the courts. Section 31(10) states that where the question of whether harm suffered by the child is significant turns on the child's health or development, his health or development shall be compared with that which could reasonably be expected of a similar child.

In Re M[13] the House of Lords, reversing the Court of Appeal, held that 'is suffering' significant harm has to be proved to be occurring at the time when the local authority began the procedure for the protection of the child, provided those arrangements have been continuously in place until the time of the hearing of the case. If the protective arrangements have been terminated, because the child's interests have been otherwise provided for satisfactorily, the test of 'is suffering' will have to be applied at the date of the hearing. The House of Lords has further decided in Re H[14] that 'likely' to suffer significant harm means a real possibility, a possibility that cannot sensibly be ignored having regard to the nature and gravity of the feared harm in the particular case. A conclusion that the child is likely to suffer significant harm must be based on facts and not just suspicion. In two more recent decisions, Lancashire C.C. v B[15] and In re O; In re B,[16] the House of Lords has grappled with the 'uncertain perpetrator' type of case where a child suffers physical harm at the hands of two or more carers but the court is unable to identify which was the perpetrator or whether all or some were perpetrators.

Part V of the Act (Sections 43–52) deals with the emergency protection of children. In particular, child assessment orders and emergency protection orders are provided. A child assessment order[17] may be made by the court, on the application of a local authority or the National Society for Prevention of Cruelty to Children (NSPCC), if it is satisfied that the local authority has reasonable cause to suspect that the child is suffering, or is likely to suffer, significant harm; and an assessment of the state of the child's health or development or the way in which he has been treated, is required to enable the local authority to determine whether or not the child is suffering or is likely to suffer significant harm. Additionally, it has to be proved that it is unlikely that such an assessment will be made, or be satisfactory, in the absence of an order. The assessment may last for a maximum period of 7 days from the date specified in the order.

The emergency protection order,[18] which replaces the place of safety order, may be granted on the application of any person who proves that there is reasonable cause to believe that the child is likely to suffer significant harm if he is not removed to accommodation provided by the applicant or he does not remain in the place in which he is then being accommodated. The order may be made for 8 days and renewed for a further 7 days.[19] It gives the applicant parental responsibility for the child. Both provisions expressly provide that a child of sufficient understanding to make an informed decision may refuse to submit to a medical or psychiatric examination or other assessment. This has been said, however, to be subject to the inherent jurisdiction of the High Court.[20]

Private law

The core of the private law provisions are contained in Part II of the Act (Sections 8–16). Section 8 orders (residence, contact, prohibited steps and specific issue) replace orders for custody or care and control and related orders. A prohibited steps order means 'an order that no step which could be taken by a parent in meeting his parental responsibility for a child, and which is of a kind specified in the order, shall be taken by any person without the consent of the court'.

A specific issue order means 'an order giving directions for the purpose of determining a specific question which has arisen, or which may arise, in connection with any aspect of parental responsibility for a child'. A prohibited steps order could, for example, be used to stop contact between a child and an 'undesirable' adult. A specific issue order may be positive or negative and its function is to regulate an aspect of upbringing.

Other provisions

Part III of the Act deals with local authority support for children and families; Part VI with community homes; Part VII with voluntary homes and organisations; Part VIII with registered children's homes; Part IX with private arrangements for fostering children; Part X with child minding and day care for young children and Part XI with the Secretary of State's supervisory functions and responsibilities. Appeals are dealt with in Section 94 and the restrictions on the use of wardship in Section 100.

Recent changes

Part 2 (Sections 111–122) of the Adoption and Children Act 2000 introduces a number of significant amendments to the Children Act 1989.[21] These cover parental responsibility of unmarried fathers, acquisition of parental responsibility by a step-parent, Section 8 orders and foster parents, the new order of special guardianship, local authority inquiries into representations, review of cases of looked-after children, advocacy services, extended meaning to 'harm' (wide supra),[12] care plans and the interests of children in proceedings.

THE HUMAN RIGHTS ACT 1998

As the courts dealing with child law have been balancing parties' rights for a long time, the introduction of the Human Rights Act 1998 has not overall had a particularly significant effect on the Children Act. The 1989 Act has generally a high degree of compatibility with the European Convention. So far, human rights law has probably had more of an impact on the decision-making process than the ultimate decisions. As the recent House of Lords case of In re S; In re W [22] shows, however, there is no room for complacency. The inability of children and parents to return to court once a local authority fails to carry out its care plan is a problem that remains to be tackled effectively. The In re S part of the case is now the subject of proceedings in the European Court of Human Rights based on arguments in respect of Articles 6, 8 and 13 of the Convention.[23]

REFERENCES AND NOTES

1. For a commentary on the Act, see The Children Act 1989 Guidance and Regulations, volumes 1–10, Department of Health 1991/92. London: HMSO.
2. Cmnd 412.
3. Chaired by the present President of the Family Division, Dame Elizabeth Butler-Sloss DBE.
4. See the Jasmine Beckford Report, London Borough of Brent, 1985; The Tyra Henry Report, London Borough of Lambeth, 1987; and the Kimberley Carlile Report, London Borough of Greenwich, 1987.
5. E.g. W v UK, 1987, 10 EHRR 29.
6. Gillick v West Norfolk and Wisbech AHA, [1986], AC 112;
7. Law Commission Working Papers No. 91; 96; 100; and 101; Report No. 100;
8. [2003], 1 FLR 210, at paragraph 73.
9. The right to respect for privacy and family life.
10. See Section 1(2).
11. See, for instance, the Protocol for Judicial Case Management in Public Law Children Act Cases, June 2003.
12. Not in force as on 26 June 2003, and no date for coming into force yet specified.
13. [1994], 2 FLR 577.
14. [1996], AC 563.
15. [2000], 2 AC 147.
16. [2003], 2 WLR 1075.
17. Section 43.
18. Sections 44 and 45.
19. But see Section 45 (2).
20. See Sections 43 (8) and 44 (7) and S. Glamorgan C.C. v B, [1993], 1 FLR 574.
21. Except for Section 116 (accommodation of children in need, etc.) not yet in force as on 26 June 2003.
22. [2002], 2 AC 291.
23. The right to a fair trial (access to court); the right to respect for privacy and family life; and the right to an effective remedy.

16

Clinical negligence

Ian Wall

Encouraged by higher expectations of healthcare provision, patients are more prepared to question their treatment, to seek explanations of adverse events, and even to embark upon litigation.

Such litigation places tremendous financial strain upon the health service,[1] as well as providing an undoubted source of stress for both clinicians and claimants alike.[2]

An individual who has suffered personal injury as a result of a medical intervention will often wish to seek some form of redress, and currently the only means of obtaining financial compensation is by pursuing an action for clinical negligence through the civil courts.

CIVIL LAW AND NEGLIGENCE

'Clinical negligence' is any litigation involving negligence in the delivery of healthcare. The law of negligence is concerned with defining the formal legal relationships that exist between private persons, where one party (the 'claimant'[3]) alleges to have been harmed by the unreasonable actions of another (the 'defendant'). The law relating to clinical negligence is a specialist area of the law of 'negligence' which itself is a branch of civil law called tort.

The principles of civil law require the claimant to discharge the burden of proving his case, by adducing sufficient factual evidence to persuade the court that it was more probable than not (i.e. greater than 50%) that the defendant's actions caused his injury.[4]

This 'balance of probability' test represents the degree of cogency or persuasiveness that is required of the claimant's evidence on the factual issues, and is known as the 'evidential standard of proof'. This standard of proof in civil cases is less onerous that the 'beyond reasonable doubt' standard employed in criminal law.

The Negligence 'Formula'

In order for an action in negligence to succeed, the claimant has to satisfy *all* the elements of a predetermined legal formula; which are that:

1 a relationship exists between claimant and defendant that gives rise to a *duty of care*,
2 this *duty of care* has, in some way, been broken or *breached* due to the unreasonable acts or omissions of the other party, (it is this breach of the duty of care that is the essence of negligence),
3 in addition, the injured party must have suffered *damage, loss* or *injury* of a type that the law recognises,
4 the defendant has *caused* this injury, and finally
5 the action has been brought within a specified time limit (the *limitation period*).

Defendants in clinical negligence

National Health Service (NHS) bodies are the usual defendants in cases of clinical negligence. They are under a direct duty to employ adequately trained professional personnel, and are 'vicariously liable' for any negligent actions (or omissions) committed by healthcare professionals in the course of their employment. As financial compensation is at the heart of an action in negligence, the NHS will also possess the necessary financial resources to satisfy any judgment against them.

Duty of care

As a general principle of the law of negligence, a duty of care is said to exist when two parties are involved in a close and proximate relationship,[5] where one party can reasonably foresee that by his action(s) (or omissions) he is likely to cause harm to the other party. Healthcare professionals and their patients clearly fall within the letter and spirit of this test.

Breach of duty and the standard of care

Where a duty has been established, parties are required to act towards one another in accordance with certain standards of conduct and behaviour. This is the 'standard of care', and in ordinary cases of negligence it is objectively calibrated by reference to what the reasonable[6] man would regard as acceptable conduct, and not *subjectively* to what the individual parties concerned consider reasonable.

Where the one party's conduct (the 'defendant's') has fallen below a minimum acceptable standard he will be regarded as being in breach of his duty towards the other (the 'claimant').

The standard of care in professionals

Healthcare workers are expected (by the courts) to exercise care and skill above and beyond that of the ordinary reasonable person. The standard governing such professional conduct is commonly referred to as the 'Bolam test', and was set down in Bolam v Friern Hospital Management Committee,[7] a case involving a plaintiff who had sustained injuries during electro-convulsive therapy. In giving judgement McNair J, made the following highly influential statement

> "The test is the standard of the ordinary skilled man exercising and professing to have a special skill. A man need not possess the highest expert skill at the risk of being found negligent. It is a well established law that it is sufficient if he exercises the ordinary skill of an ordinary man exercising that particular art. "

This aspect of the test is a recognition of the logic that increased skill imposes increased duties.

McNair J continued further, stating that a practitioner;

> "is not guilty of negligence if he had acted in accordance with a practise accepted as proper by a responsible body of medical men skilled in that particular art."

This element of the test, approved by the House of Lords in Maynard,[8] provides the practitioner with a 'defence' to an allegation of clinical negligence, so long as he is able to demonstrate that his conduct is supported by a body of responsible opinion (even if a body of opinion also exists that is critical of the conduct in question). This test of 'acceptable practice' has attracted criticism as it, in effect, allows the medical profession to set both the factual and legal limits of their duties, a situation which often presents an insurmountable hurdle to claimants. The Bolam test was born of an age when the courts appeared to exhibit a considerable degree of deference to specialist areas of medical decision-making.

Recently, however, the courts have adopted a more critical approach to the conclusiveness of peer-opinion, and appear prepared to analyse the logic behind a particular medical practice, and decide for themselves whether the practice was reasonable.[9]

A variable standard

The issue of how the standard of care should be reflected in the various strata of medical experience and expertise was examined in Wilsher v Essex *AHA*.[10] The case involved a junior and 'inexperienced' doctor who had incorrectly inserted an umbilical catheter into a pre-term baby in order to monitor the oxygen concentration in the blood. Unsure as to the catheter's position he sought the advice of his registrar, who was of the erroneous opinion that the catheter was indeed correctly sited.

As a consequence of this error, the infant received excessive quantities of oxygen, which, it was later contended, caused him to develop blindness. In giving judgement, the Court of Appeal was mindful of balancing training requirements in hospitals with patient protection, and acknowledged that too high a standard may discourage practitioners from entering specialist areas, while one set too low would afford a ready 'defence' of inexperience.

In rejecting the notion of a standard tailored to the experience of an individual practitioner, the court concluded that the standard should reflect the post occupied by the practitioner and that the standard that of an averagely competent and well-informed practitioner who fills a post in a unit offering a highly specialised service.[11]

SPECIFIC BREACHES OF DUTY

In practice, healthcare professionals undertake a multiplicity of activities, all with attendant legal duties.

A doctor has a duty to attend and treat his patients; he will not automatically be liable for an incorrect diagnosis, but he will be expected to arrive at the diagnosis with due care and skill, missing only conditions that any other reasonably competent practitioner would also fail to diagnose.[12]

It is the duty of the doctor to keep up with advances in medical practice. He is, however, not required to have an exhaustive knowledge of recent advances and is not under a duty to put into operation all the suggestions of contributors to medical journals, unless they are standard practice.[13]

A doctor has a duty to communicate to his patient any risks (but not all) involved in treatment,[14] to refer to a specialist, and arrange diagnostic tests when appropriate.

In private medicine, a practitioner may also be liable to his patient in contract,[15] for breach of an implied contractual term to provide his services with due skill and care. In rare circumstances the practitioner has even been regarded as having guaranteed that his treatment would succeed.

DAMAGE

Proof that damage, i.e. actual loss or injury, has occurred is vital in cases of negligence, as the law does not hold actionable so-called 'negligence in the air'. An individual practitioner may embark upon a careless or inadvertent course of action but, provided it does not cause any injury, there is no liability. The damage, furthermore, must be of a nature or type that is recognised by the law as actionable.

CAUSATION

Causation is the connection between the negligent act and the damage or injury suffered by the claimant.

Causation is often the sole area of contention in a case of clinical negligence, as the defendants often concede issues of 'duty' and 'damage'. In order to succeed on the issue of factual causation the claimant has to show that;

> **but for** the defendant's fault (or negligent act), on the balance of probability, the injury complained of (or the 'gist' of the damage) would not have occurred.

In Barnett v Chelsea and Kensington Hospital Management Committee[16] the defendant's employee, a doctor, in breach of his duty had declined to attend a patient who, unbeknown to all, had been the victim of a poisoner. In the civil action that followed the patient's death, the plaintiff's representative failed the 'but for' test. The court established that by the time the patient had arrived at the hospital his fate was sealed, even if the defendant had provided appropriate treatment the plaintiff would have perished.

The 'balance of probability' is the standard of proof on the factual issues, so that a claimant, to be successful, must demonstrate a statistical likelihood of greater than 50% that the defendant caused the injuries complained of.

In 'simple' cases, where the medical and scientific evidence is clear and uncontroversial, the issue of causation poses little practical or conceptual difficulty. Clinical interactions are, however, often complex, and expert medical evidence on factual issues is often not amenable to the type of statistical interpretation preferred by lawyers. The medical evidence may suggest an association or *casual* link between insult and injury, but this may not be sufficiently cogent to support a *causal* link. This often presents insurmountable problems for claimants, especially where more than one causative agent is implicated in the genesis of an injury.

In order to address some of the complexities associated with 'causation', the courts may, under certain circumstances, be moved to bridge this 'evidential gap' by inferring causation as a matter of law.

Both the plaintiffs in Bonnington Castings v Wardlaw[17] and McGhee v NCB[18], suffered injury as a result of exposure to a harmful environmental agent from two different sources, one of which ('the guilty agent') was a consequence of the negligence of the defendants who employed them. In both cases, the plaintiffs' failure to satisfy the 'but for test', due to the inherent deficiencies in the state of contemporary medical knowledge, was mitigated by the court which held that they could succeed if it could be shown that the guilty agent had 'materially contributed' to the injury[17] or the *risk* of injury.[18]

In Wilsher, however, The House of Lords declined to extend this line of inferential reasoning, which permitted the separation of guilty and innocent components of one possible causative agent, into situations where the defendant's actions had merely added (excess oxygen) to a number of possible causes of the injury complained of (prematurity, brain haemorrhages of, hypoxia).

LOSS OF A CHANCE

The 'but for' test is an all or nothing test, so that provided the defendant's negligence does not create a risk greater than the background risk he will not be liable, and damages will not be awarded.

In Hotson v East Berkshire AHA[19] the claimant, a 13-year-old boy, fractured his femur in a fall; an injury that was missed in the course of the defendant's negligent mismanagement. The plaintiff subsequently suffered a recognised complication of this injury that, even with appropriate management, he stood a 75% of developing.

Under these circumstances, the plaintiff would fail the 'but for' test as the background risk of developing the complication was greater that 50%, and accordingly he would not receive damages.

In order to circumvent this hurdle, the 'gist of the damage' was reformulated into the 'loss of a chance', that is, the loss of the prospect of a better clinical outcome. The defendant's negligence now rested on the proposition they had converted the plaintiff's 75% probability of developing the complication into a 100% certainty, or put another way, the defendant's negligence meant that the plaintiff's chance of *not* developing the complication was reduced from a 25% chance to a zero chance. This contention initially found favour with the Court of Appeal but was subsequently rejected by the House of Lords.

DAMAGES

Damages are the pecuniary award for injuries suffered and 'quantum' is the financial measure of this. The general aim of damages in tort is to put the injured party, so far as is possible, into the position he would have been in if the tortuous act had not been committed and the claimant had not been injured.

As such, the injured party must be compensated for any pain and suffering arising from the injury itself, as well as any financial losses that may be incurred as a result of a reduced capacity to compete in the employment marketplace. In addition, monetary compensation is awarded to ensure that there are sufficient funds to provide for any future medical care.

LIMITATION PERIOD

Limitation periods exist to encourage speedy claims and to prevent the undue hardship of indefinite litigation, not least for the practical difficulties involved in adducing and interpreting stale evidence.

The Limitation Act 1980 (Section 11) imposes a time limit of three years on claimants bringing an action for negligence resulting in personal injury, and any claims outside this period will be barred.

The clock starts to run from the date at which the action accrued, or alternatively the time when the claimant knew, or ought reasonably to have known, the facts giving rise to the action were the result of a negligent action by an identifiable defendant (Section 14).

The court maintains a jurisdiction to override the limitation provisions in exceptional cases if, having regard to all the circumstances, it would be equitable (fair) to do so.[20]

If at the time of the injury a person is under 18 years of age, then the limitation period does not begin (i.e. the cause of action does not accrue) until they attain majority, or if mentally ill until they recover (Section 28).

HEALTHCARE AND CRIMINAL LAW

There has been an increased willingness by the criminal justice system to undertake the prosecution of doctors whose patients die as a result of their mistakes, as a series of high profile cases concerning spinal administration of cytotoxic drugs testify.[21]

In R v Adamoko[22] the Court of Appeal stated that a jury should only convict in circumstances of 'gross negligence', where there is a serious breach of duty and a serious departure from a proper standard of care, and where, by his actions, the practitioner has exhibited a disregard for the life and safety of others.

CIVIL PROCEDURE

The Woolf Report[23] sought to address widespread criticism of the process of civil litigation with its impenetrable rules, and endemic problems of delay[24] and excessive costs.[25] This systemic examination, and the resulting legislation which implemented many of the Report's recommendations,[26] attempted to remedy the stale, rule bound ethos of civil justice in the UK.

The civil courts now operate under an overriding objective to deal with cases 'justly', and are tasked with 'active case management', in order to ensure a timely and expeditious resolution of disputes. A 'tracking' system has been introduced which reflects variations in complexity and financial value between cases.[27]

In addition 'pre-action protocols' or directions have been introduced, specifically directed at the parties to clinical disputes.[28] This protocol is designed to ensure that issues are identified at an early stage in the litigation process, to facilitate communication, and to focus the attention of litigants on the desirability of resolving disputes without resorting to formal litigation.

A key feature of the new system is an explicit awareness that the courtroom may not always be the appropriate arena in which to resolve disputes. Consequently, considerable emphasis is placed on alternative dispute resolution and independent mediation, supported rather pragmatically by financial incentives for early settlements (CPR Part 26 and 36).

Detailed 'protocol' procedure seeks a timed sequence of formal contact between the litigants, efficient exchange of relevant documentation, as well as provisions for mutually agreed expert reports (though little used).

A DIFFERENT SYSTEM

The current system of 'blame-based' litigation has been criticised as fundamentally flawed[29] as its punitive approach acts as a disincentive to open admission and reporting of 'significant' events.

Despite the procedural changes introduced following the 'Woolf Report' the civil litigation system still remains costly and time consuming with lawyers often being the main beneficiaries. There has been periodic consideration of the merits of introducing a 'no-fault' compensation scheme in the UK.[30] Such a system is founded on principles of proof of injury rather than proof of fault so that claimants would be compensated regardless of whether there had been negligence.[31]

No-fault schemes have attracted the attention of the current UK government as a means of addressing the burgeoning costs of servicing clinical negligence claims. Most recently, however, the Chief Medical Officer[32] has rejected a comprehensive no-fault system on the grounds, paradoxically, of excessive cost and has instead favoured a tariff and tribunal model akin to the Criminal Injuries Compensation system.

PAYING FOR JUSTICE

The principle of providing access to justice for those of 'slender means' in the form of state-funded legal aid, traces its origins to the post war welfare state ideals.

Escalating costs in the provision of this service led to systemic reforms[33] in which the Legal Services Commission replaced the old legal aid scheme and certain categories of cases were excluded from receiving legal aid. In addition, the scope of conditional fees, so called 'no win no fee' (where lawyers receive no fee if a case is lost) was extended.

REFERENCES AND NOTES

1. In 1974–1975 annual NHS clinical negligence expenditure was GBP 1 million (GBP 6.33 million at 2002 prices). According to the National Audit Office some 10,000 new claims were received in the period 1999–2000 costing nearly GBP 400 million with liabilities relating to unsettled cases at GBP 2.6 billion, and a further GBP 1.3 billion relating to un-reported cases; Report by the Comptroller and Auditor General HC 403; 'Handling Clinical Negligence Claims in England'. HC 403. The Stationary Office, London (www.nao.gov.uk). For 2001–2002 the annual clinical negligence expenditure was GBP 446 million.
2. An Organisation with a Memory, Department of Health 2000. The Stationary Office (www.doh.gov.uk/cmo/orgmem/).
3. The 'claimant' will bear the burden of proof under the doctrine 'he who asserts must prove'. The term 'claimant' replaced 'plaintiff' following the introduction of the CPR (26). Older cases retain their original nomenclature but the two are interchangeable.

4. *Cassidy v Ministry of Health*, 1951, 2 KB 343.
5. This relationship is referred to as the 'neighbour' test initially formulated in *Donoghue v Stevenson*, 1932, AC 562.
6. The reasonable man was the legal fiction referred to as the man on the Clapham Omnibus. He is the ordinary man, whose fictional perspective acts as an objective fixed point when judging conduct in court, thereby introducing a degree of consistency between various judgements.
7. *Bolam v Friern Hospital Management Committee*, 1957, 2 All ER 118. See also infra Consent to Medical Treatment where the judgement in Bolam is employed in assessing 'best interests' and 'necessity of treatment,' as well as 'sufficiency of information.'
8. *Maynard v West Midlands Regional Health Authority*, 1984, 1 WLR 634.
9. *Bolitho v City and Hackney Health Authority*, 1993, 4 Med LR 381 (CA), where Dillon LJ introduced Public Law notions of reasonableness laid down in *Associated Provincial Picture Houses Ltd. v Wednesbury Corporation*. Unreasonableness in this context relates to conduct and decisions that defy logic.
10. *Wilsher v Essex Area Health Authority*, 1987, QB 730 CA; 1986, 3 All EWR 800; 1988, AC 1074 (HL).
11. per Mustill LJ at (1986) 3 All ER 800 at 812.
12. Misdiagnosis is the most frequently alleged incident in case of clinical negligence.
13. *Crawford v Board of Governors of Charing Cross Hospital*, *The Times* 8 December 1953.
14. *Infra*; Chapter on Consent to Medical Treatment.
15. *Thake v Maurice*, 1986, 1 All ER 499.
16. 1969, 1 QB 428.
17. *Bonningtons Castings v Wardlaw*, 1956, 1 AC 613 (HL).
18. *McGhee v NCB*, 1972, 3 All ER 1008.
19. *Hotson v East Berkshire AHA*, 1987, AC 750 (HL).
20. In exercising this power the court will look at such matters as the length and reason for the delay, and the conduct of both parties Under S33 Limitation Act 1980.
21. *R v Prentice*; *R v Suliman*, 1993, 3 WLR 927, defendants both junior doctors convicted but acquitted on appeal. Drs Dermott Murphy and John Lee (case dropped by Crown Prosecution Service).
22. *R v Adamoko*, 1991, 2 Med LR 277.
23. The Final Report on Access to Justice in 1996.
24. Average time to settle currently 5 1/2 years after receipt of the claim. Report by the Comptroller and Auditor General HC 403; 'Handling Clinical Negligence Claims in England' *ibid*.
25. In the period 1999–2000, 65% of the settlements below £50,000, legal and other costs involved in settling the claim exceeded the damages awarded, Report by the Comptroller and Auditor General HC 403; 'Handling Clinical Negligence Claims in England'.
26. 1997 Civil Procedure Act and the 1998 Civil Procedure Rules.
27 Civil Procedure Rules 1998 SI 1998 No. 3132 R 1.4.
28. Pre-Action Protocol for the Resolution of Clinical Disputes: www.lcs.gov.uk/civil.

29. Lord Kennedy in the Report on the Inquiry into the management of care of children receiving complex heart surgery at the Bristol Royal Infirmary. Command Paper: CM 5207. See earlier chapter on Legal Systems and Public Enquiries. (www.bristol-inquiry.org.uk.)

30. No-fault compensation schemes currently operate in New Zealand and Scandinavian Countries, though the experiences there are not readily transferable to the UK.

31. No-fault compensation schemes currently operate in the UK in the form of the Industrial Injury Scheme, the Criminal Injuries Compensation Scheme, and the Vaccine Damage Payment Scheme.

32. The proposed NHS Redress Scheme: Making Amends – a consultation paper setting out the proposals for reforming the approach to clinical negligence in the NHS; a report by the Chief Medical Officer, DOH, June 2003.

33. Access to Justice Act 1999, which followed the Woolf Report.

17

Legislation for medicines and product liability

Robin Harman

INTRODUCTION

All medicines for human use are subject to stringent legislative controls before any product can be sold or supplied for use by health professionals and patients. The need for legislation to ensure that extensive testing of products is carried out before medicinal products are marketed was prompted by the teratogenic effects produced by thalidomide. The limb deformities produced by the drug would have been detected in the reproductive toxicology tests now routinely required during the drug development programme.

Today, medicinal products can only be supplied once their quality, safety, and efficacy have been assessed by the Licensing Authority and a marketing authorisation (previously called a product licence) has been issued. Current procedures by which a marketing authorisation is obtained are laid down in, primarily, European Union (EU) legislation. The legislation comprises Regulations, which are directly applicable in all Member States; Directives, which must be transposed into national legislation prior to implementation; and guidelines, which have no legal status, but which a manufacturer wishing to place a product on the market has to give good reasons for not following.

The complexity and scope of information that must be generated before in a marketing authorisation application can be submitted is shown in Table 17.1.

One of the major problems with legislation is that it rarely remains unchanged for any length of time. This is especially true for legislation affecting medicinal products because of the advances in science and technology with which legislation tries to keep up. Modifications to legislation for pharmaceuticals continue to be proposed and made. Significant proposals are currently under discussion, with their final implementation likely in 2004.

Product liability is a complex issue when applied to medicinal products. Medicines are given to patients with the expectation that the product will

Table 17.1 Presentation of the marketing authorisation application.

The marketing authorisation application (MAA) consists of administrative information and the necessary demonstration of quality, safety, and efficacy of the product. This is presented in four parts:

Part I	*Summary of the Dossier*
Part IA	Administrative data
Part IB1	Summary of product characteristics (SPCs)
Part IB2	Proposal for packaging, labelling, and package insert
Part IB3	SPCs already approved in the Member States
Part IC	Expert reports
Part IC1	Expert report on the chemical, pharmaceutical, and biological documentation
Part IC2	Expert report on the toxico-pharmacological (preclinical) documentation
Part IC3	Expert report on the clinical documentation
Part II	*Chemical, pharmaceutical, and biological documentation*
Part IIA	Composition
Part IIB	Method of preparation
Part IIC	Control of starting materials
Part IID	Control tests on intermediate materials
Part IIE	Control tests on the finished product
Part IIF	Stability
Part IIG	Bioavailability/Bioequivalence
Part IIH	Data related to the environment risk assessment for products containing genetically-modified organisms (GMOs)
Part IIQ	Other information
Part III	*Toxico-pharmacological documentation*
Part IIIA	Toxicity
Part IIIB	Reproductive function
Part IIIC	Embryo-foetal and perinatal toxicity
Part IIID	Mutagenic potential
Part IIIE	Carcinogenic potential
Part IIIF	Pharmacodynamics
Part IIIG	Pharmacokinetics
Part IIIH	Local tolerance
Part IIIQ	Other information
Part IIIR	Environment risk assessment
Part IV	*Clinical documentation*
Part IVA	Clinical pharmacology
Part IVB	Clinical experience
Part IVQ	Other information

produce some benefit. However, risks are also inherent in their administration, and it is necessary to achieve a balance between the benefits and
risks. The condition for which the medicine is being used will influence
the risk:benefit ratio or therapeutic index. For relatively minor conditions (e.g. a headache or short-term diarrhoea), only a small degree of
risk will be tolerated, requiring a large therapeutic index. For more serious conditions (e.g. cancer or heart failure), the medicines used may be
potentially more harmful, but their use is tolerated because of the severity of the condition being treated.

CONTROL OF MEDICINES

Early UK legislation

In the UK, the Medicines Act was given Royal Assent in October 1968,
consolidating and expanding existing, but inadequate, legislation and
became operative on 1 September 1971. It covered all aspects of the
development, manufacture, packaging and labelling, distribution, and
advertising of medicinal products for human and veterinary use. It put
on a statutory footing the activities of the former Committee on Safety
of Drugs for human medicinal products. Separate bodies cover veterinary
medicines, but are not considered in this Chapter.

The Medicines Act created the Medicines Commission, which advises
the UK regulatory authority for human medicines, the Medicines and
Healthcare Products Regulatory Agency (MHRA), and Ministers (the
Licensing Authority) on matters relating to medicinal products. The
Medicines Commission in turn advises on the setting up of specialist
committees, which currently comprise:

- Advisory Board on the Registration of Homoeopathic Products
- British Pharmacopoeia Commission
- Committee on Safety of Medicines (which superseded
  the Committee on Safety of Drugs)
- Veterinary Products Committee

The CSM has established three subcommittees to support its work:

- Chemistry, Pharmacy and Standards
- Biologicals
- Pharmacovigilance

More recently, two further committees have been set up:

- Independent Review Panel for Advertising
- Independent Review Panel on the Classification of Borderline
  Substances

The Medicines Commission and the above 'Section 4 Advisory Committees' (formed under Section 4 of the 1968 Medicines Act) must be consulted before a decision is taken by the Licensing Authority to refuse a marketing authorisation application. They must also be consulted should it be necessary to revoke, vary, or suspend a marketing authorisation on grounds of quality, safety, and efficacy.

Early European legislation

Running in parallel to the introduction of the Medicines Act in the UK was the development of a legislative framework in Europe. This has had an increasingly important influence on the control of medicines in the UK, especially from the early 1990s onwards. The first legislation adopted by the then six members of the European Economic Community (EEC) was Directive 65/65/EEC, and this still forms the basis for existing legislation today. The UK joined the EEC in 1973, and the second phase of EEC legislation for pharmaceuticals was adopted in 1975.

Directive 75/319/EEC initiated the programme to create a single market in pharmaceuticals. A Committee for Proprietary Medicinal Products (CPMP) was formed to help Member States agree to decisions relating to medicines' control. A new procedure to assess and approve marketing authorisations was also established, initially called the CPMP procedure and later renamed the multi-state procedure. This was intended to minimise duplication of the assessment procedures for marketing authorisation applications in different countries and to promote a harmonised market for pharmaceuticals throughout Europe. However, there was a marked reluctance by Member States to agree to others' assessments and almost all applications had to be referred to the CPMP for arbitration.

At the same time, Directive 75/320/EEC established a Pharmaceutical Committee, with a membership from all Member States, to advise the European Commission on policy matters relating to medicinal products.

In 1987, a further authorisation procedure was introduced by Directive 87/22/EEC, termed the concertation procedure. Its use was mandatory for biotechnology products and optional for high-technology products. Member States could consult each other when carrying out the assessment of these complex medicines, and the new system proved moderately successful.

Concurrent to the changes to the major legislation affecting marketing authorisations, the European Community (EC) (as it had by then become) generated a considerable number of other Directives that affected all Member States, including the UK. These covered all aspects of the marketing of medicinal products for human use.

Current UK and European legislation

Neither the multi-state nor concertation procedures proved as successful as had been hoped. As a result, a major review of approval procedures was started in the late 1980s and resulted in what was then called the 'Future Systems' package. This comprised:

- EC Regulation 2309/93, which established a new European regulatory authority, the European Agency for the Evaluation of Medicinal Products (EMEA) and a new centralised procedure for obtaining a marketing authorisation (see below)
- Directive 93/39/EEC for human medicinal products, which amended Directives 65/65/EEC, 75/318/EEC, and 75/319/EEC
- Directive 93/41/EEC which repealed Directive 87/22/EEC.

The 'Future Systems' legislative package came into effect on 1 January 1995 and is the basis of the current system of approval of medicinal products in the UK and the rest of the EU. Under the legislation, medicinal products can be authorised by one of two means.

The centralised procedure

The centralised procedure, established by Regulation 2309/93, is compulsory for biotechnological medicinal products and optional for new chemical entities. It is possible that its use may become mandatory for all new chemical entities under the ongoing review of legislation (see below). The assessment of the marketing authorisation application is carried out by the EMEA, who nominates a rapporteur and co-rapporteur (both from the members of the CPMP) to oversee the assessment. If approved, the authorisation issued by the European Commission is automatically valid across the entire EU.

The mutual recognition procedure

The mutual recognition procedure is controlled by Directives 93/39/EEC (for human medicines) and 93/40/EEC (for veterinary medicines) and by Regulation 541/95 (used for varying the terms of marketing authorisations). Under the mutual recognition procedure, one of the EU national regulatory authorities (the Reference Member State) undertakes the assessment of the marketing authorisation application. If approved, a national marketing authorisation is issued. The details of the authorisation are then sent to other 'Concerned Member States' in which the pharmaceutical company wishes to market the product. These Concerned Member States are intended to mutually recognise the authorisation.

Application of the new EU legislation in the UK

The UK Medicines Act was not deemed suitable for transposing many of the new European Directives (the EU Regulation was automatically effective in all Member States). As a result, new UK legislation was promulgated, called The Medicines for Human Use (Marketing Authorisations Etc.) Regulations 1994, which became effective on 1 January 1995. The UK Regulations provided legislation that cross-referred to the European legislation rather than setting out the texts in full. This method of implementation was chosen to minimise the duplication of UK and EU law, to ensure that the EU law was implemented in full, and to minimise potential complications when later changes were made to EU legislation.

In essence the UK Medicines for Human Use (Marketing Authorisations Etc.) Regulations 1994 provide the following controls:

- the requirements for marketing authorisation applications and the procedures for granting, varying, and renewing marketing authorisations
- obligations imposed upon UK marketing authorisation holders, including pharmacovigilance requirements
- labelling and package leaflet requirements
- provisions relating to the Licensing Authority to suspend, compulsorily vary, or revoke a marketing authorisation
- related enforcement measures

Framework legislation for pharmaceuticals

The most important legislation that has been introduced in the EU, and which has direct relevance to UK legislation, is listed in Table 17.2.

Review of pharmaceutical legislation

Table 17.2 shows that a great number of Directives and Regulations have been introduced and implemented over a number of years into which inevitably inconsistencies were introduced. To overcome this, the legislation was recast into a single legislative text, Directive 2001/83/EC for human medicinal products, which is termed the Community Code and which supersedes all the previous texts.

In 1995, it had been agreed that a review of the new systems would take place after 5 years in operation, and the review of pharmaceutical legislation was started in 2000. The proposed changes are a consequence of the enlargement of the EU in 2004–2005 to 25 Member States and of the experience gained by using the systems as they were implemented.

Table 17.2 Important legislation for medicinal products for human use in Europe.

Directives

65/65/EEC	On the approximation of provisions laid down by law, regulation or administrative action relating to medicinal products
75/318/EEC	On the approximation of the laws of Member States relating to the analytical, pharmacotoxicological and clinical standards and protocols in respect of testing of medicinal products
75/319/EEC	On the approximation of provisions laid down by law, regulation or administrative action relating to medicinal products
89/105/EEC	Relating to the transparency of measures regulating the pricing of medicinal products for human use and their inclusion within the scope of national health insurance schemes
89/342/EEC	Extending the scope of Directives 65/65/EEC and 75/319/EEC and laying down additional provisions for immunological medicinal products consisting of vaccines, toxins, or serums and allergens
89/343/EEC	Extending the scope of Directives 65/65/EEC and 75/319/EEC and laying down additional provisions for radiopharmaceuticals
89/381/EEC	Extending the scope of Directives 65/65/EEC and 75/319/EEC and laying down additional provision on the approximation of provisions laid down by law, regulation or administrative action relating to proprietary medicinal products and laying down special provisions for medicinal products derived from human blood or human plasma
91/356/EEC	Laying down the principles and guidelines of good manufacturing practise for medicinal products for human use
92/25/EEC	On the wholesale distribution of medicinal products for human use
92/26/EEC	Concerning the classification for the supply of medicinal products for human use
92/27/EEC	On the labelling of medicinal products for human use and on package leaflets

(continued)

Table 17.2 (*continued*).

Directives

92/28/EEC	On the advertising of medicinal products for human use
92/73/EEC	Widening the scope of Directives 65/65/EEC and 75/319/EEC on the approximation of provisions laid down by law, regulation or administrative action relating to medicinal products and laying down additional provisions on homoeopathic medicinal products
93/39/EEC	Amending Directives 65/65/EEC, 75/318/EEC, and 75/319/EEC in respect of medicinal products
93/41/EEC	Repealing Directive 87/22/EEC on the approximation of national measures relating to the placing of high-technology medicinal products, especially those derived from biotechnology
2001/83/EC	On the Community Code relating to medicinal products for human use

Regulations

EEC 2309/93	Laying down Community procedures for the authorisation and supervision of medicinal products for human and veterinary use and establishing a EMEA
EC 297/95	On fees payable to the EMEA
EC 540/95	Laying down the arrangements for reporting suspected unexpected adverse reactions which are not serious, whether arising in the Community or a third country, to medicinal products for human or veterinary use authorised in accordance with the provisions of Council Regulation (EEC) No 2309/93
EC 541/95	Concerning the examination of variations to the terms of a marketing authorisation granted by a competent authority of a Member State
EC 542/95	Concerning the examination of variations to the terms of a marketing authorisation falling within the scope of Council Regulation (EEC) No 2309/93
EC 1662/95	Laying down certain detailed arrangements for implementing the Community decision-making procedures in respects of marketing authorisations for products for human or veterinary use

Proposed changes to the EMEA

The structure of the Agency and its Committees is to be changed. The CPMP is to be renamed the Committee for Human Medicinal Products (CHMP); representation from each Member State on the Committees is to be reduced; and the Agency's Management Board is to be restructured. A new Committee of Herbal Medicinal Products is to be formed to work alongside the CHMP, the Committee for Veterinary Medicinal Products (CVMP), and the Committee on Orphan Medicinal Products (COMP).

Proposed changes to the centralised procedure

It has been proposed to broaden the scope of the procedure so that it is mandatory for all new chemical entities. Other proposals shorten the time allowed for assessment of applications, the introduction of fast-track procedures for major innovative products, removing the 5-year expiry date for authorisations, and increasing the number of safety reports that the company holding the authorisation has to produce.

Proposed changes to the mutual recognition procedure

The timescale for carrying out the assessment of an application is to be reduced from 201 days to 150 days, and the legislative framework for postmarketing pharmacovigilance is to be strengthened so that urgent action by one Member State must be implemented at a Community level.

THE MHRA

The Licensing Authority for the UK comprises the Ministers in the Department of Health. The Ministers are accountable to Parliament on matters relating to human medicines' regulation in the UK. Medicines are controlled by a system of licensing and conditional exemptions from licensing as laid down in UK and EU legislation.

Up to April 2003, authorisations to manufacture, market, distribute, sell, and supply medicinal products were granted in the UK by the Medicines Control Agency (MCA) on behalf of the Licensing Authority. The MCA was an Executive Agency of the Department of Health. (Medicines can also be authorised by the centralised procedure (see above) for which the Licensing Authority is the European Commission.)

In April 2003, the MCA and the UK authority responsible for controlling the quality and safety of medical devices, the Medical Devices Agency (MDA), were combined into a single authority, the MHRA. The reasons for this move were to centralise the licensing processes for all human healthcare products and to reflect the trend towards an increasing number of products manufactured that comprise both a medicinal product and a medical device.

The MHRA is self-funding, being supported by the fees it charges industry and others for the services it provides. The Secretary of State for Health holds responsibility for the activities of the MHRA and is accountable to Parliament for its activities.

The MHRA controls clinical trials, advertising and other promotional claims, quality control, manufacture of products that do not have a marketing authorisation, and the supply of imported medicinal products. The safety of medicinal products that have a marketing authorisation is also controlled (pharmacovigilance), and the MHRA is required to take action when adverse effects occur with authorised medicinal products. The MHRA is also the UK Good Laboratory Practice Monitoring Authority.

PRODUCT LIABILITY

A medicinal product is manufactured under closely controlled conditions and granted a marketing authorisation with approved indications for its clinical use. Problems in the use of medicines can arise from a number of causes:

- the manufacturing process or the conditions in which the medicine is stored may be inadequate, leading to products of defective quality;
- the prescriber or pharmacist may inadvertently supply a product for an inappropriate use or may give inappropriate instructions for its safe use;
- the patient may use the medicine incorrectly causing unintended or intended harm.

In only the first instance does the question of strict product liability come into effect. However, the other examples can equally cause harm and have been the source of legal actions to determine 'cause' and 'liability'.

It is also important to stress that the incidence of cases of product liability is relatively small and has not mirrored the explosion of litigation in other areas of healthcare. This may be a consequence of the strict controls imposed upon the manufacture and supply of medicinal products;

or may be due to the difficulty that is sometimes experienced in identifying where strict liability for a fault actually lies.

Legislation covering product liability

The product liability Directive (Directive 85/374/EEC) was implemented into UK law by the Consumer Protection Act 1987. The Directive
provides for strict liability against the supplier of a defective product.
A defective product is defined as one which does not provide the safety
a person is expecting when the presentation of the product, its use, and
the time at which the product was made available have been taken into
consideration. From the perspective of medicines, a product cannot be
deemed defective just because an improved product has become available. If the product was manufactured according to the then current
'state of the art', this is a defence against strict liability.

The Directive renders liable the manufacturer of the product.
Irrespective of whether the product is a proprietary medicinal product
or a generic product, the manufacturer is the legal entity who leads others
to understand that he is the producer of the medicine.

Manufacturing issues

Very tight legislative controls are maintained at all stages in the manufacture and distribution of medicines. This is codified by Good Manufacturing
Practice and Good Distribution Practice and a system of licensing for manufacturing, wholesaling, and importation (e.g. Directive 91/356/EEC).
Controls range from monitoring the quality of starting materials and the
need for full documentation for all manufacturing activities, to the impos-
ition of long-term (usually more than 2 years) storage conditions and the
information leaflets that are supplied with the medicine.

The MHRA Inspection and Enforcement Division has a statutory
responsibility to ensure that the highest possible standards have been met
during manufacturing and distribution of medicines. The Inspections
Group in the Division inspects all manufacturing facilities every 2 years.
Inspection of wholesale premises is carried out every 4 years.

The Division also runs a Medicines Testing Scheme. Each year, it
takes about 2000 largely randomly chosen samples of both licensed and
unlicensed medicinal products for analysis, mainly from community
pharmacies.

The Defective Medicines Reporting Centre (DMRC) at the MHRA
receives about 150 reports of defective products each year and issues
drug alerts as required. These potential quality defects are submitted by

Table 17.3 Examples of defects reported by the Defective Medicines Reporting Centre (DMRC) at the MHRA in 2002/3.	
Product	Reason for recall
Diazepam 10 mg/2 mL injection	Two batches recalled as visible particles detected in several batches after 2 years of storage
Crisantapase 10,000 units/ vial	All batches recalled as a precautionary measure following an in-depth review of process revalidation results relating to sterility assurance
Carbimazole 20 mg tablets	Two batches may contain up to one-fifth sub-potent tablets, containing up to 50% lower than the specified strength
Salbutamol 100 µg/inhalation inhaler	Three batches recalled as faulty valve may lead to up to 3–5 times the expected dose being delivered
Diltiazem 240 mg capsules	One batch recalled as some of the 240 mg capsules have been packaged in blisters intended for 180 mg strength capsules

the public, professional bodies, and pharmaceutical companies. Examples of defects reported in 2002–2003 are listed in Table 17.3.

Prescribing problems

The diagnosis made by a doctor in the consulting room, or by a pharmacist when undertaking 'counter-prescribing' of non-prescription medicines, may be incorrect. As a result, an inappropriate medicine may be supplied either on prescription or through a sale direct to the patient. The prescriber may also elect to prescribe a product for an indication for which the medicine has not been approved ('unlicensed use'). In such cases, the liability for the use of the product rests with the prescriber rather than with the manufacturer.

This 'unlicensed use' is a particular problem with the treatment of children's illnesses. Most of the medicines approved for adult use have not been tested for use in children. One reason for this is the high cost of conducting clinical trials in a separate age-group which is less likely to be recouped through the relatively small potential market for children's medicines. Moreover, the definition of 'children' provides a far from homogeneous group, ranging from neonates and infants to adolescents, further complicating the conduct of clinical trials.

Issues associated with use by patients

Directive 92/27/EEC requires that all medicines are supplied with a patient information leaflet that has been approved by the regulatory authority at the same time as the marketing authorisation. The information in the patient leaflet is intended to be written in an understandable and straightforward manner. Despite the value of providing patients with information about the medicine they are taking, several problems co-exist. One is the requirement that they list all possible side-effects and adverse events that might arise. The scale and scope of such information may be off-putting to many patients, making them less likely to start or complete treatment.

Medicines may be administered by patients themselves or by medical staff on their behalf. Again, while not strictly a product liability issue, medication errors that occur may be caused by a number of factors. Issues that might have indirect product liability implications include labelling, the packaging, and the name of the product. The errors may be related to the prescribing, dispensing, or administration of the product.

The former absence of a central reporting system for medication errors in the NHS resulted in the same errors being repeated many times in different locations. One attempt to resolve this issue was the creation in the UK in July 2001 of the National Patient Safety Agency (NPSA). The NPSA, a Special Health Authority of the NHS, was set up to promote patient safety by creating a national reporting system across the NHS for adverse events and near misses, designing solutions that prevent harm, and promoting research into patient safety issues.

Two of the common causes of errors are the similarity of drug names and confusion with strengths of the same drug. Examples include the trade names Losec and Lasix; amiloride 5 mg and amlodopine 5 mg; atenolol 50 mg and atenolol 100 mg; and co-codamol 8/500 and co-codamol 30/500.

Dispensing errors that occur relate to supply of the incorrect product or an incorrect strength of the correct drug. Giving the incorrect dosing instructions on the label and affixing the wrong label to the product are two other significantly harmful problems. The risks associated with the use and misinterpretation of abbreviations when prescribing or dispensing are also major concern in trying to minimise medication errors.

REFERENCES AND FURTHER READING

The Rules governing medicinal products in the European Union
Volume 1: Pharmaceutical legislation - medicinal products for human use.
Volume 2A: Notice to Applicants - medicinal products for human use.
Volume 2B: Notice to Applicants - medicinal products for human use.
Volume 3A: Guidelines - medicinal products for human use - quality and biotechnology.
Volume 3B: Guidelines - medicinal products for human use - safety and the environment.
Volume 3C: Guidelines - medicinal products for human use - efficacy and information on the medicinal product.
Volume 4: Good manufacturing practices - medicinal products for human and veterinary use.
Volume 5: Pharmaceutical legislation - medicinal products for veterinary use.
Volume 6A: Notice to Applicants - medicinal products for veterinary use.
Volume 6B: Notice to Applicants - medicinal products for veterinary use.
Volume 7A: Guidelines - medicinal products for veterinary use - safety and the environment.
Volume 7B: Guidelines - medicinal products for veterinary use - efficacy and information on the medicinal product.
Volume 8: Maximum residue limits - medicinal products for veterinary use.
Volume 9: Pharmacovigilance - medicinal products for human and veterinary use.

All: Luxembourg, Office for Official Publications of the European Communities, 1998.

18

Clinical trials: ethical, legal and practical considerations

Christobel Saunders

Much basic medical research is carried out in laboratories. However, new diagnostic and therapeutic measures eventually need to be tested on humans – first by studying drug delivery and toxicity in healthy volunteers, then drug efficacy and activity in a limited group of patients – Phase I and Phase II studies. Following these studies a new treatment must be tested against conventional therapy by means of the Phase III study or randomised controlled clinical trial (RCT). Finally, on-going surveillance of treatments is carried out either by individual doctors and institutions auditing results or by reporting of adverse events. For example in the UK, since 1964, doctors have been asked to report suspected adverse drug reactions to the Medical and Healthcare Regulatory Agency through a Yellow Card scheme.

This chapter will concentrate on the randomised clinical trial and examine some ethical, legal and practical considerations of conducting or participating in clinical trials.

The RCT was first developed by RA Fisher in the 1920s for agricultural research, and was introduced some 20 years later into medicine in a trial evaluating antibiotic treatment for tuberculosis.[1] An RCT is a study in which a cohort of subjects with a defined disease is randomly allocated to one or other treatment (which may be an established *versus* either a new treatment, or using a placebo drug as the control) and their outcomes recorded. Randomisation aims to avoid the types of bias inherent in observational studies, such as confounding, which may result in apparent differences between treatment groups which do not in fact exist.

By recruiting large numbers of subjects to a trial the chance that the outcomes between the two arms will differ because of unequal distribution to risk factors becomes small. It is possible to calculate this probability – the p-value.

If a trial is designed to encompass any patients with a given condition the results can be generalised to the prevention or treatment of the disease as a whole.

Ethical issues

Ethics provide a pathway of reasoning whereby a morally respectable and defensible position can be reached.[2] A doctor's first duty is always said to be to his patient, thus he may face an ethical dilemma when wishing to enter a patient into a clinical trial in which the treatment will be allocated randomly.[3] Equally the patient faces the ethical challenge of relinquishing autonomy. Both parties are in effect putting the greater good of society ahead of the individual to ensure future generations of patients receive the best possible treatment.

However a number of arguments can be forwarded to soften this position. Firstly if the doctor (and thus by extension the patient) does not know which treatment will be best (i.e. is in equipoise) offering a patient entry into a trial of treatments may be most fair. Secondly it can be argued that not only does the doctor have a duty to undertake research but that the patient also has a duty to participate in clinical trials, as his treatment is a result of previous patients' contribution to medical science.

Clinical trials raise a number of problems for both the 'trialist' (i.e. the doctor) and the 'subject' (i.e. the patient). A doctor who participates in research must always put the good of the individual patient above the pursuit of knowledge. The patient expects that his doctor will first and foremost protect and promote his welfare. Yet the clinician may be genuinely uncertain as to the best possible form of treatment and so wish to enter his patient in a trial. He must then randomise the patient's treatment and may use a placebo. Explaining these issues to the patient may weaken the doctor-patient relationship – so often based upon the belief that 'the doctor knows best'.

If a patient does agree to enter a clinical trial it must be without coercion for consent to be valid. In practise this may be hard to achieve as many patients feel they must agree to anything to 'please the doctor'.

International guidelines

The attention of the medical community, and indeed the world, was first focused on the issue of the ethics of human experimentation following the disclosure of Nazi practises during World War II. In 1946, at the trial of 23 German doctors charged with 'war crimes' and 'crimes against humanity' for their experimentation on prisoners of war and civilians, the Nuremberg Code was established.[4] This aimed to protect the interests of human participants in research. Building upon this, the World Medical Assembly in 1964 adopted the Declaration of Helsinki containing 'recommendations guiding physicians in biomedical research involving human subjects'.[5] This was most recently adopted at the 52nd World Medical Association General Assembly in 2000.[6]

These guidelines recommend that a patient should firstly be assured of the best proven diagnostic or therapeutic method, and that any new treatment being tested will be *at least* as advantageous as any other, with a reasonably low chance of side-effects. The patient must be informed of the benefits and hazards of all possible treatments, and must be free to refuse to participate in a trial or withdraw at any time. The physician must also be free to change to another treatment if he feels this will benefit the patient. The patient may also anticipate that the doctor/investigator will keep any excess investigations in the trial to a minimum.

A number of other international agencies are involved in research guidelines: the International Conference on Harmonisation (ICH) of Technical Requirements for Registration of Pharmaceuticals for Human Use[7] attempts to bring together regulatory authorities and pharmaceutical experts from Europe, Japan and the US to harmonise scientific and technical aspects of product registration. Many individual countries have developed their own comprehensive guidelines for clinical research: in the US the National Committee for Quality Assurance and the Joint Commission on Accreditation of Healthcare Organisations[8] have collaborated to form the Partnership for Human Research Participation, which accredits institutions, has a national set of standards and a voluntary oversight process that complements current regulatory efforts; in Australia the Therapeutic Goods Administration has developed a document pertaining to the regulation of clinical trials[9] to complement existing regulation of new drugs through the Clinical Trials Notification (CTN)/Clinical Trial Exemption (CTX) schemes; in South Africa a national set of research guidelines exists.[10]

In the UK a number of medical bodies have also developed guidelines. These include the Medical Research Council (MRC), the Royal College of Physicians, the Kings Fund, the British Medical Association, the Medical Sterile Products Association and the Association of the British Pharmaceutical Industry (ABPI). There is no statutory legislation on human experimentation (except the Human Fertilization and Embryology Act 1990), however pharmaceuticals are regulated via the Medical and Healthcare Regulatory Agency (MHRA) which was formed from a merger of the Medicines Control Agency and the Medical Devices Agency in April 2003. It is expected this body will help steer the new European Directive on Good Clinical Practice in Clinical Trials.[11]

Consent

To allow a patient to express his autonomy, he must be fully informed about his disease and its treatment. This will include details of the clinical trial he is being requested to join, along with the risks and benefits of all possible treatments (of course a patient outside a trial should also be informed of all possible treatments and not only the one he is offered). If he then consents to the treatment or trial this may be said to be informed consent (see also Chapter 5).

The MRC in its 1986 document 'Responsibility in investigations on human subjects' states that:

> in general, patients participating in RCTs should be told frankly that different procedures are being assessed and their cooperation invited. Occasionally, however, to do so is contraindicated.[12]

Thus we are faced with another dilemma – although it is ethically imperative to obtain a patient's fully informed consent before initiating any treatment within a clinical trial, it appears that there may be situations in which full disclosure is harmful to the patient.[13] This predicament has been shown to be a major factor in poor accrual rates into clinical trials.[14] The issues of gaining consent in special circumstances such as the unconscious patient, for minors or in the mentally ill, is beyond the scope of this chapter.

The ethics of good science

To undertake a study which is not likely to answer the scientific question posed is not only bad science but unethical: the patient is being subjected to tests or treatments, the efficacy of which cannot be proven in the study. To overcome this, major funding agencies and many ethical committees insist that any proposed research is carefully scrutinised by peer review processes.

The design and delivery of clinical trials has thus become a discipline unto itself, which calls on the skills of a wide range of scientists, clinicians, biostatisticians, data managers and many others. Within this discipline there are many controversies which include an ethical component such as inclusion criteria, protocol deviation, conflicts of interest and issues related to privacy (which in the UK is guided by the 1998 Data Protection Act and the EU data protection directive 95/46/EEC). Another example of this are the stopping rules for clinical trials.

In the design of a study, rules are written which allow an independent data-monitoring group to stop the trial if adverse outcomes exceed pre-set limits. For example, in May 2002 an arm of the Women's Health Initiative Study[15] was stopped 4 years early because these stopping rules were breached. In this study otherwise well older women were randomised to receive Hormone Replacement Therapy (HRT) or a placebo, the hypothesis being that HRT would prevent a number of diseases including heart disease. In fact a little over half way through follow up it was found that there was an excess of heart disease (as well as excess breast cancer and stroke, a more expected outcome) and that this very small increase had exceeded the stopping rules. Ethically the trial monitors had to stop the study – it appeared that women in the study were getting more heart diseases, not less, as a result of taking HRT, although there were no excess deaths recorded. However many clinicians and scientists in the field were disappointed, as stopping the trial early has meant we will never know if taking HRT makes women more likely or less to die from heart disease, and it is unlikely we will ever again be able to repeat this kind of study.

Ethics committees

Virtually all institutions involved in patient care, and many health-related organisations, have ethics committees (or institutional review boards in the US). These committees are tasked with reviewing applications for research projects on human subjects, and can look at a wide range of aspects from the science of the project, to its ethical viability to practical aspects such as whether the institution and researchers have the facilities and expertise to undertake the treatment proposed. A detailed description of the work of these committees can be found on the Central Office for Research Ethics Committees website (www.corec.org.uk).

LEGAL ISSUES

The Medicines Act 1968 regulates approval of all new drugs (See Chapter 10). However in the UK there is currently no legislation specifically governing the conduct of clinical trials either of drugs or medical and surgical therapies, although this may develop from the European Directive on Good Clinical Practice in Clinical Trials.

Legal discussion regarding clinical trials, as well as standard treatment, has mainly centred around the issue of consent. Lord Scarman has said, 'If a patient is fit to receive information and wishes to receive it, the doctor must 'brief' the patient so he can make a free and informed choice'.[16]

How much information should be given to the patient to allow him to make an informed choice, however, is open to interpretation and thus dissention. From an ethical standpoint there is a spectrum of views, ranging from those whose first concern is patient autonomy and full disclosure to those who adopt a paternalistic viewpoint in which the doctor must judge how much information he feels his patient requires, depending upon factors such as personality and perceived ability to understand information, the nature of the treatment and the magnitude of possible harm.

If a patient feels he has suffered harm as a result of being subjected to a treatment he may choose to bring charges of negligence. He must prove that the doctor failed to provide sufficient information regarding the treatment and that this failure has caused him harm as he would not have consented to the treatment if full information had been given.

Many feel that the current state of the law fails to reflect full patient autonomy, although as Kennedy confirms,[3] there is in fact no law relating directly to clinical trials.

In the case of healthy volunteers in drug trials, the Association of the British Pharmaceutical Industry has issued guidelines concerning compensation.[17] The Consumer Protection Act 1998 states that a pharmaceutical company is liable for compensation for injury caused by a defective drug, and most pharmaceutical company sponsored trials will offer ex-gratia compensation schemes. However it can be contested,[18,19] that there is need for some form of no-fault compensation procedure in all clinical trials, irrespective of whether or not they are run by a drug company, so that the burden of proving causation does not fall on the patient. It should be the responsibility of ethics committees who review research protocols to ensure this compensation is allowed for.

What is the likely outcome today for a patient who feels he has not been properly informed of some aspect of his treatment within a clinical trial? Kennedy[3] suggests that the courts would try to ensure that a patient has given informed consent and would use the doctor's evidence for this. In the course of treatment outside a clinical trial, if a doctor felt he had a compelling reason *not* to disclose fully all information this would almost certainly be accepted, in the UK at least, as being in the patient's best interests. Within a trial, it is accepted that there must be disclosure to a patient firstly that he is in a clinical trial, secondly all the associated risks of the 'new' treatment, plus a doctor must answer honestly any questions posed to him by the patient. Furthermore, 'Even if a certain risk is a mere possibility that ordinarily need not be disclosed, yet if its occurrence raises serious consequences, as for example paralysis or even death, it should be regarded as a material risk requiring disclosure'.[3]

PRACTICAL CONSIDERATIONS

To be ethically and legally sound a clinical trial protocol must be based upon solid scientific design, preferably an *a priori* hypothesis and good clinical practice. It must be performed by an experienced investigator and must have undergone review by an independent ethics committee. Much research will also have been peer-reviewed as part of a funding process.

Incorporation of the patient preferences into the design of trials may mean an alteration, for example in the type of patient recruited or the inclusion of a non-randomised arm, but bears consideration if we wish to incorporate the whole community in research.[20]

A trial, whether run by a pharmaceutical company or a research institution, must be regularly monitored by an independent body to ensure that there is no misconduct, and that one arm of the study is not prematurely showing a significant beneficial or harmful outcome. This usually means setting up an independent data monitoring committee. Equally a mechanism must exist to report and act on any side effects reported, and if necessary stop the trial.

The investigator must ensure he obtains fully informed consent, preferably in written form. Such consent should include the purpose of the trial, the benefits both to the patient and to the society, any possible risks and alternative treatments, and the right to refuse or withdraw at any time. The patient should understand that results of the trial will be published, although he may be reassured that confidentiality will not be breached. The concepts of uncertainty and randomisation should be explained. The use of patient information sheets, closely scrutinised by an ethics committee is encouraged.

It is important that patients are not coerced into entering trials; thus payment should not be offered in treatment trials, and healthy volunteers may only be paid a relatively modest sum. The use of 'captive audiences' in trials – such as medical students or prisoners – is controversial, although it may be said that any patient asked to enter a clinical trial by the doctor treating him feels under some obligation to comply to please the doctor.

Finally in the analysis of the trial data, good practice such as intention to treat analysis should be adhered to, and publication of results sought. The Consolidated Standards of Reporting Trials (CONSORT) statement[21] aims to improve reporting of trials and facilitate their inclusion into systematic reviews, and is mindful of ethical issues.

SUMMARY

Is the goal of achieving certainty via the RCT too high a price to pay in ethical terms? Should we perhaps concentrate further on obtaining data from observational studies and other methods?

This author believes that well-conducted randomised clinical trials continue to provide the best quality of data and offer the patient a fair plan of treatment. This can be further improved by good communication between the health workers and the patient including the use of counsellors, written information and interactive videos. Involving patients in the organisation of clinical trials and educating them to demand the best treatment, including treatment within a trial, should go hand in hand with educating doctors at undergraduate and postgraduate levels about the ethical, legal and practical issues involved in research.

Although the ethics of clinical experimentation have been widely debated, the legal standpoint awaits clarification until suitable cases have been brought to the courts. Perhaps it would be reasonable to conclude that the consequences, both ethical and practical, of not performing proper RCTs trials are too alarming to contemplate.

REFERENCES AND FURTHER READING

1. British Medical Journal (author anonymous), 1948, Streptomycin treatment of pulmonary tuberculosis: a Medical Research Council investigation. *Brit. Med. J.* 2: 769–782.
2. Ward CM, Ethics in surgery. *Ann. Roy. Coll. Surgeons Eng.*, 1994, 76: 223–227.
3. Kennedy I. Consent and randomised clinical trials. In: Kennedy I 1988 *Treat Me Right*. Oxford: Clarendon Press, 1988.
4. US Government, Trials of war criminals before the Nuremberg military tribunal under Control Council law, 1949, US Government printing office, Washington DC.
5. World Medical Assembly, 1964, Declaration of Helsinki. Recommendations guiding medical doctors in biomedical research involving human subjects. (Adopted by the 18th World Medical Assembly, Helsinki, Finland 1964.)
6. World Medical Assembly, 2000, Declaration of Helsinki, amended by the 52nd World Medical Assembly, Edinburgh, Scotland, 2000.
7. International Conference on Harmonisation of Technical Requirements for Registration of Pharmaceuticals for Human Use. www.ich.org
8. National Committee for Quality Assurance and the Joint Commission on Accreditation of Healthcare Organisations. www.jcaho.org
9. Regulation of Clinical Trials in Australia. TGA, May 2002. www.health.gov.au/tga/

10. Guidelines for Good Practice in the Conduct of Clinical Trials in Human Participants in South Africa. http://196.36.153.56/doh/docs/policy/trials/trials_01.html

11. European Directive on Good Clinical Practice in Clinical Trials. http://www.mca.gov.uk/ourwork/licensingmeds/types/clintrialsbriefnote.pdf

12. Medical Research Council. Responsibilities in investigations on human subjects. London: Medical Research Council, 1986.

13. Saunders CM, Baum M, Haughton J. Consent, research and the doctor–patient relationship. In: Gillon R (ed.) *Principles of Health Care Ethics*. Chicester: Wiley, 1994.

14. Taylor KM, Margolese RG, Soskoline CL. Physicians' reasons for not entering eligible patients in a randomised clinical trial of surgery for breast cancer. *New Eng. J. Med.*, 1984, 310: 1363–1367.

15. Writing Group for the Women's Health Initiative Investigators. Risks and benefits of Estrogen plus Progestin in healthy postmenopausal women principal results from the women's health initiative randomized controlled trial. *JAMA*, 2002, 288: 321–333.

16. Scarman L. Consent, communication and responsibility. *J. Roy. Soc. Med.*, 1986, 79: 697–700.

17. Association of the British Pharmaceutical Industry. *Guidelines for Medical Experiments in Non-Patient Human Volunteers*. Association of the British Pharmaceutical Industry, London, 1988.

18. Brazier M. *Medicine, Patients and the Law*, 2nd edn. London: Penguin, 1992.

19. Mason JK, McCall Smith A. *Law and Medical Ethics*, 4th edn, London: Butterworths, 1991.

20. Lambert MF, Wood J. Incorporating patient preferences into randomized trials. *J. Clin. Epidemiol.*, 2000, 53: 163–66.

21. www.consort-statement.org

19

Medicolegal implications of blood-borne viruses

Felicity Nicholson

INTRODUCTION

Medical conditions may have direct medicolegal implications. This chapter explains in detail the background to blood-borne viruses in terms of incidences and impact from a medicolegal perspective. The serendipitous discovery, by Blumberg 1965, of the so-called Australia antigen (now known as hepatitis B surface antigen) and its association with serum hepatitis heralded the dawn of a new era – the recognition that blood and/or other body fluids can transmit infection. Since then there has been an increased awareness amongst healthcare professionals and lay people alike about infections from other blood-borne viruses (BBVs) – Hepatitis D Virus (HDV), the Human Immunodeficiency Virus (HIV) and Hepatitis C Virus (HCV) – and their potentially fatal complications. Doctors have a duty of care to their patients, to educate and wherever possible treat such infections. They also need to prevent the spread of infection by protecting others who might be placed at risk. In some situations issues of consent and confidentiality may arise leading to ethical dilemmas.

In 1889 the Infectious Disease (Notification) Act was introduced in England and Wales to identify and prevent the spread of infectious diseases. Over time certain diseases were eradicated and others were added. The Public Health (Control of Diseases) Act 1984 requires the statutory notification of cholera, plague, relapsing fever, small pox, typhus and food poisoning. A further 24 diseases are required under the Public Health (Infectious Diseases) Regulations, 1988. The latter includes all forms of viral hepatitis but not HIV, which has led to difficulties in monitoring the prevalence and epidemiology among the population.

This chapter describes the individual viruses in chronological order, gives data on global and UK prevalence and highlights population subgroups at specific risk. It also includes the development of international and European legislation pertaining to BBVs and the way the law has intervened on the legal rights and duties of medical personnel and infected individuals to protect others and prevent the spread of such viruses, most notably HIV.

OVERVIEW OF THE INDIVIDUAL BBVs

Hepatitis B virus

An estimated 2000 million people have been infected with Hepatitis B Virus (HBV) worldwide and of those more than 350 million have chronic infection – a condition that can lead to cirrhosis, and/or liver cancer and renders them potentially infectious to others. Globally, HBV kills about one million people per annum. Since 1982, a safe and effective vaccine has been available which is 95% effective in preventing infection and its long-term sequelae. In 1992, the World Health Organization (WHO) recommended that hepatitis B vaccine should be integrated into the national immunisation programmes by 1995 of all countries whose chronic infection rate was 8% and into all countries by 1997.

By the end of 2001, 135 countries had achieved this goal. Unfortunately, the countries with the highest prevalence are also the poorest and cannot afford it. The Global Alliance for Vaccines and Immunisation (GAVI, created in 1999) and the Global Fund for Children's Vaccines have been striving to change this. HBV can be transmitted by a variety of routes as shown in Table 19.1.

HBV can also be a risk for healthcare professionals – the risk of acquiring the virus from a single needle stick exposure varies from 1–30% depending on the level of infectivity of the contact. In industrialised countries (e.g. Western Europe, North America, Australia and New Zealand)

Table 19.1 Routes of HBV transmission.

- Perinatal (from mother to baby either before or during birth)
- Unprotected sexual contact (homosexual/heterosexual)
- Percutaneous exposure to blood or bloodstained body fluids through unsafe injections, unsafe transfusions, unsafe surgical/dental procedures and tattooing
- Unsafe organ donation
- Penetrating bite injuries whether or not blood is involved
- Other mucocutaneous exposure – eye, mouth
- Contamination of fresh wounds, 24 hrs old with blood or other body fluids
- Prolonged and close personal contact – household settings, institutionalised patients.

all personnel have to be vaccinated before commencing medical prac-tise. These same countries also encourage and help other at-risk groups to be vaccinated (e.g. police officers, workers in care homes and prisons, homosexual/bisexual men and Intravenous Drug Users (IVDUs)). Again, Healthcare Workers (HCWs) born and working in countries with the high-est prevalence (e.g. China, the Indian sub-continent and Sub-Saharan Africa) and others who are at-risk are the least likely to be protected.

HDV

HDV, a defective single-stranded RNA virus requiring hepatitis B for repli-cation, was discovered in 1977. It has a varied clinical course ranging from an acute self-limited infection to fulminant liver failure. Approximately 15 million people are infected worldwide. The global pattern of HDV cor-responds with the prevalence of chronic HBV. In countries where chronic HBV infection is low, HDV occurs mainly among IVDUs, people receiving multiple blood transfusions and among haemophiliacs. In countries with moderate or high prevalence of chronic HBV the prevalence of HDV is highly variable. In southern Italy and parts of Russia and Romania HDV prevalence is high, occurring in >20% of asymptomatic HBV carriers and >60% of patients with HBV-related chronic liver disease. Other areas with a high prevalence include North Africa and the Middle East, the Amazon basin and the American South Pacific Islands of Samoa, Hauru and Hiue. Strangely, in China and most of Southeast Asia, where HBV prevalence is high, infection with HDV is rare.

Infection can be acquired either as a co-infection with HBV or as a superinfection of a person with chronic HBV infection. Co-infection often leads to a more serious acute illness and a higher risk of fulminant disease than with HBV alone. However, chronic HBV infection is less likely to develop when infection with HDV is simultaneous (<5% of patients). Superinfection with HDV, however, is more likely to lead to chronic liver disease with cirrhosis (70–80%) than among patients with chronic HBV alone (15–30%).[1] It also has a greater risk of developing fulminant hepatitis in the acute phase (compare 1% in co-infection with 5% in superinfection).

The modes of transmission for HDV are similar to hepatitis B, with percutaneous exposure being the predominant route. It is particularly prevalent in IVDUs. Sexual transmission of HDV is less efficient than HBV and perinatal transmission is rare. A person is only infectious when hepatitis Delta antigen or HDV RNA is present in serum. These markers are present in the acute phase of the illness, but may persist if chronic infection occurs. This is more likely in the case of superinfection.

Preventing HBV by vaccination will obviously help to eliminate the chance of acquiring HDV by co-infection. For those already infected with HBV, the only way of preventing superinfection with HDV is by educating the individuals concerned about reducing risk behaviours.

Interferon-alpha (e.g. Roferon) is used to treat patients with chronic HBV and HDV infection. There is some indication that using a higher dose may be more successful in eliminating both viruses.[2,3]

HIV

In 1981 attention was drawn to two publications in the Morbidity and Mortality Weekly Report of the Centers for Disease Control (Atlanta, Georgia, USA) of a potentially new immunosuppressive disease that appeared to be targeting homosexual men. This arose from a sudden increase in the number of reports of *Pneumocystis Carinii* Pneumonia (PCP) and Kaposi's sarcoma amongst gay men in San Francisco, Los Angeles and from New York City.[4,5] And so began the hunt to find the causative agent. In 1983, the combined efforts of two eminent physicians, Robert Gallo in America and Luc Montagnier in France, finally identified a new human retrovirus, now known as HIV.

Following intensive research it became apparent that the virus had been in existence probably since the late 1960s in Africa, but no one could have predicted the devastating worldwide implications of this infection.

A report from WHO prepared in collaboration with Joint United Nations Programme on HIV/AIDS (UNAIDS) – The AIDS Epidemic Update December 2002 (Table 19.2) revealed that to date some 42 million adult and children are infected with HIV/AIDS, with 5 million new infections in 1 year. Table 19.2 shows the distribution by region, the percentage prevalence in adults, women, and the main modes of transmission. More than 80% of the worlds total, live in Africa and India. However, a recent report in The Lancet[6] suggests that China could face a similar explosion of HIV as India unless rapid action was taken to control the spread of HIV-1. By the end of 2001, the UN estimated that between 800,000 and 1.5 million were already infected and numbers could reach 10 million by 2010.[7] The majority of infections are attributable to intravenous drug use and transfusions of infected blood and blood products,[8] but sexual transmission may become the predominant route as the virus spreads from IVDUs and sex workers in to the general population.

The first case of AIDS in the UK was reported in 1982 and all clinicians in England and Wales were encouraged to inform the Communicable Disease Surveillance Centre (CDSC) at Colindale and in Scotland to the Scottish Centre for Infection and Environmental Health of other likely

Table 19.2 WHO data in collaboration with UNAIDS. The AIDS Epidemic Update November 2002.

Region	Epidemic started	Adult + child HIV/AIDS	Adult − child newly infected	Adult prevalence %	% HIV + +ve women	Main mode transmission
Sub-Saharan Africa	Late 70s early 80s	29.4 million	3.5 million	8.8	55	Heterosexual
N Africa Middle East	Late 80s	550,000	83,000	0.3	55	Hetero IVDU
S and SE Asia	Late 80s	6 million	70,000	0.6	36	Hetero IVDU
E Asia + Pacific	Late 80s	1.2 million	270,000	0.1	24	IVDU
						MSM
						Hetero
Latin America	Late 70s early 80s	1.5 million	150,000	0.6	30	MSM
						IU
						Hetero
Caribbean	Late 70s early 90s	440,000	60,000	2.4	50	Hetero
						MSM
E Europe + Central Asia	Early 90s	1.2 million	250,000	0.6	27	IVDU
W Europe	Late 70s early 80s	570,000	30,000	0.3	25	MSM
						IVDU
N America	Late 70s early 80s	980,000	45,000	0.6	20	MSM
						IVDU
						Hetero
Australia + NZ	Late 70s early 80s	15,000	500	0.1	7	MSM
Total		42 million	5 million	1.2	50	

cases. Reporting had to be and still is confidential. With the advent of antibody testing in 1984 (HIV-1) and 1985 (HIV-2) it became easier to monitor the spread of infection. Results from diagnostic testing (voluntary testing with informed consent) may be unrepresentative and could either over- or underestimate the true prevalence.[9,10]

Similarly mandatory testing of blood donors also underestimates population prevalence by excluding those most at risk of infection. Voluntary unlinked surveillance using blood specimens left over from diagnostic testing for other purposes was then introduced, but too many participants declined for the tests to be carried out, rendering the data hard to interpret. This led to much consideration and debate as to how to ensure that HIV was monitored in a way that was both legal and ethical.[11]

Finally in 1990 integrated national unlinked anonymous (blinded) surveillance programmes were introduced and are still in place. The statistics obtained help in devolving budgets to specific high-risk populations and areas of higher prevalence. However, they will never be wholly reliable as underreporting of new cases and duplication of reports may occur.

In the UK cumulative data to the end of December 2002 reported 54,261 individuals with HIV/AIDS (including AIDS related deaths). The group identified at greatest risk of acquiring HIV are homosexual/bisexual men. 28,835 of the cumulative total fell into this category.[12] The next most significant group are IVDUs. The risks from blood, blood products and organ donation have been drastically reduced since the introduction of routine screening for HIV and improvement in viral inactivation techniques. In 1992 The European Collaborative Study published data in The Lancet[13] indicating that the risk of transmission in Western Europe was 14%. Other studies conducted in Africa painted a different picture with transmission rates up to 45%.[14,15] The higher rates were attributed to mothers having a greater viral load and concomitant placental infections rendering the placenta more permeable to the virus. Since then the use of anti-viral treatment during pregnancy has led to a startling decrease in transmission risks. Data from a randomised, controlled clinical trial conducted by the Pediatric AIDS Clinical Trials Group (PACTG 316) was published in July 2002.[16] It used a two-dose nevirapine regimen (one dose given to the mother during labour and another to the child within 72 hours of delivery alongside maternal treatment during pregnancy with Zidovudine (AZT), AZT/3TC or other drug combinations) and showed an overall HIV transmission rate of 1.5%. However, the reality is that countries with the highest transmission rates are also the poorest and drug treatment is rarely available.

The estimate of HIV transmission after a single percutaneous exposure (calculated from reported worldwide data available) is 0.32% (22/6955), and from a mucocutaneous exposure −0.03% (1/2910).[17]

Table 19.3 Summary of routes of HIV transmission with percentage risk.

- Homosexual/bisexual men – figure unknown but still group at greatest risk
- IVDUs – 1% overall (3.5% in London)
- People from endemic areas (>80% of world total from Africa and India)
- Babies of HIV +ve mothers. Without treatment 14% in Europe and up to 45% in Africa
- People receiving unscreened blood transfusions or blood products

HCV

HCV was first identified in 1989 and was recognised as the major virus responsible for non-A non-B transfusion hepatitis. Since then, six genotypes and more than 50 subtypes of HCV have been recognised. According to the WHO it is now a global public health problem with some 3% of the population having been infected.[18] This means that more than 170 million people are chronic carriers of the virus and are at risk of infecting others.

Prevalence of the virus varies from country to country and within a given country according to risk group. In about 10% of acute cases of hepatitis C and 30% of chronic cases, the source of infection is unknown. Such infections are called sporadic or community-acquired infections. However, for many countries what little data exists is often unreliable. This is largely due to the different generations of screening assays used.

The highest prevalence exists in Egypt (17–26%). This has been ascribed to contaminated needles used in the treatment of schistosomiasis carried out between the 1950s and the 1980s.[19] Intermediate prevalence (1–5%) exists in the Mediterranean, Eastern Europe, the Middle East, the Indian subcontinent and parts of Africa and Asia. In Western Europe, most of Central America, Australia and limited regions in Africa including South Africa the prevalence is low (0.2–0.5%). Previously America had been included in the low prevalence group, but a more recent report[20] indicates that almost 4 million Americans (1.8% of the population) have antibody to HCV, representing either ongoing or previous infection. It also states that HCV accounts for approximately 15% of acute viral hepatitis in America.

Studies in the UK, conducted on blood donors, suggest that the overall prevalence is 0.5%. High-risk groups include haemophiliacs who received blood products prior to 1984, when inactivation of blood and blood factors was introduced to reduce the risk of HIV. Of those still alive almost 100% have been infected. Currently the greatest risk comes from IVDUs with prevalence estimates between 46% and 90%. The variation in the figure reflects in part, the length of time that an individual has been injecting. (The longer the time, the greater the risk.) A recent study of 3000 current IVDUs recruited from the community and from treatment agencies showed an overall prevalence of 30%.[21] However, this is likely to be an underestimate as those at greatest risk are less likely to seek help.

The risk among homosexuals/bisexuals and regular heterosexual partners of infected individuals (with no other risk factors) is <5%, indicating that the predominant mode of transmission is through blood. The risk to babies of infected mothers is around 6% and transmission is thought to occur around the time of delivery. Breast-feeding is not considered a risk to the newborn unless the mother is also infected with hepatitis B and/or HIV.

Most people who contract HCV remain asymptomatic during the acute phase of the illness, and are therefore unaware that they are infected. Eighty per cent of those with detectable HCV antibodies have HCV RNA in their blood rendering them infectious to others. This makes the spread of HCV difficult to control except through increasing awareness among the general population of how the virus is transmitted.

The Department of Health (DoH) document 'Hepatitis C Strategy for England'[22] states that 80% of infected individuals will develop chronic infection, 75% of these will get some form of liver damage and inflammation, and 20% develop cirrhosis. Also there is approximately a 2% (1.25–2.5%) chance of patients with cirrhosis, secondary to HCV, developing hepatocellular carcinoma. Factors leading to an increased risk of developing rapid and severe liver disease include:

- Acquisition of HCV over the age of 40
- Male
- Alcohol consumption

By the end of 1990 screening tests for HCV antibodies became available in some laboratories in the UK. Positive tests were confirmed by the Public Health Laboratory Services, CDSC based at Colindale. By 1993 nearly all Public Health Laboratories in England and Wales were performing anti-HCV Elisa tests. Blood donations have been screened for HCV since 1991. Current estimates for England suggest that the risk of an HCV infectious donation entering the blood supply is >1 in 200,000.[23]

Cumulative data collected to the end of December 2001 have reported 26,500 infections in England. This is about 10% of the number of infections estimated from seroprevalence studies, reflecting that the majority of cases remain undiagnosed.

The importance of recognising infection at an early stage allows advice about changes in lifestyle to be given (e.g. reducing alcohol intake) and the possibility of a combination treatment of Ribavirin and interferon alpha-2b or one of the newer pegylated interferons.[20]

THE ROLE OF INTERNATIONAL LAW

HIV has had more impact on international and, indeed, national law than any other BBVs. The question is why? It is not about numbers, since HIV has approximately 1/50th of the worldwide prevalence of hepatitis B. More likely reasons are that at the start of the epidemic HIV/AIDS was classified as a fatal disease and was initially associated with certain risk behaviours that led to discrimination. Also the introduction and increasingly widespread use of an effective vaccine in 1982 for hepatitis B has helped to limit the spread of infection.

Whatever the explanation, since its emergence in the early 1980s, HIV/AIDS has demonstrated the different levels on which the law can operate. These can be divided into three categories or models: proscriptive, protective, and instrumental.[24]

The proscriptive model

The proscriptive impact of the law became apparent early on in the HIV epidemic because of the particular epidemiology of HIV infection in developed countries. Homosexual men and injecting drug users were identified as the highest risk groups in the West. In many jurisdictions in America, for instance, such behaviours constituted a criminal offence. Criminal sanctions were also imposed in Ireland for buying condoms[25] and in Australia, workers in needle-exchange programmes feared prosecution for aiding and abetting an illegal activity, or for 'possession' in the form of traces of illegal drugs remaining in the used needles and syringes.[26] Proscriptive laws have also impacted in a much broader context in developing HIV strategies. For example, laws for compulsory reporting of HIV positive individuals, laws requiring the testing of certain population groups, such as prisoners[27] and immigrants[28] and laws that compel disclosure of a person's HIV status under certain circumstances. Instead of reducing or limiting the spread of infection these laws had the reverse effect, as the people most at risk were discouraged from identifying themselves. Such people are also likely to be characterised by socio-economic disadvantage and discrimination. It is ironic that those countries where most new cases occur are also the ones that have been unable to stop or even reduce the rate of infection.

The protective model

This aspect of the law endeavours to protect individuals or groups of people from harmful and undesirable occurrences. It has played a central role in acting to preserve individual rights and prevent the discrimination as demonstrated above. At the heart of this, lies the International Human Rights Law developed after the Second World War and the formation of the United Nations in 1945. They apply to every individual irrespective of gender, religious beliefs, and nationality and are intended to protect the civil and political rights, to prevent private sector discrimination and preserve the right to health. The ability of a given state to impose limitations on certain personal freedoms (e.g. the right to liberty of movement) must adhere to a set of established rules. It has to be lawful, and be the least intrusive and least restrictive and achieve the specific interest in a democratic society.[29]

For protective laws to be effective they must include a proscriptive element that imposes penalties for non-compliance. However, the main aim is still to protect the individual from unnecessary discrimination and thus to encourage responsible behaviour without fear of redress. The proscriptive element has to be included for the 'greater common good'. Sometimes it may be necessary for an individual's rights to be breached to protect others. In particular this may apply to the issues of confidentiality and disclosure of HIV status where a healthcare professional may legitimately inform a patient's sexual partner of their HIV status.[29] In 2002, the High Commission for Human Rights and UNAIDS revised the 6th guideline to ensure that domestic legislation was flexible enough to promote and ensure access to HIV/AIDS prevention, treatment, care and support for all.[30]

While the International Guidelines on HIV/AIDS and Human Rights addresses the member states' moral responsibility to affected people, it plays no part on a personal obligation.

The instrumental role

This is the most controversial model for legal intervention and also the most difficult to interpret and apply. Its approach looks beyond the rights of the individuals to endeavour to change the underlying values and patterns of social interaction to reduce the risk of HIV to the most vulnerable. This approach became apparent in the early years of the epidemic when western countries concentrated on civil and political rights to prevent discrimination against those with HIV/AIDS and to protect the individual's liberty.

In developing countries, where the major route of HIV transmission was through heterosexual intercourse and from mother to baby, these attitudes were considered narrow-minded and unrealistic. They were more concerned with socio-economic and developmental rights. It is important, therefore, that human right approaches should take all factors into account when developing public health policies.

Emphasis has also been placed on ensuring that member states should ensure community consultation in all phases of HIV/AIDS policy design, programme implementation and evaluation, the aim being to prevent individual governments from introducing laws and policies that increase inequality and discrimination, resulting in further HIV infection.

AUTONOMY IN EUROPEAN LAW

In the beginning there was much argument across Europe on the appropriate response to manage and control the spread of HIV infection. Only two jurisdictions in Western Europe (Bavaria and Sweden) chose to use the proscriptive approach.

In Bavaria routine compulsory testing for sex workers, non-European immigrants and new entrants to the civil service was introduced. Gay clubs and saunas were closed. Contact tracing was instigated and infected people were barred from certain forms of employment. Those who failed to comply were detained and isolated.

In 1985 Sweden included HIV among the venereal diseases covered by the Communicable Diseases Law, 1968. This allowed infected people to be registered, their contacts traced, and patients behaving in a way that could spread the disease to be isolated. People testing HIV positive must undergo regular medical examinations, and inform all previous sexual partners and doctors and dentists treating them. The police can also be involved to deal with anyone failing to comply with these regulations.[31] Hofmann in 1988 stated that these policies involved 'a massive abridgement of the fundamental right of free movement, the general right of personality and the human dignity of the affected person'.[32]

The rest of Western Europe took the reverse approach by encouraging individuals to protect themselves and therefore others. Health education campaigns were established to condition behaviour by highlighting the risk of infection and how such risks could be reduced. This enabled the autonomy of the individual to be preserved. These measures were supplemented by the intervention of gay activists who played a prominent role in countering panic, resisting coercion and in developing an autonomy-focused response to the spread of AIDS in certain parts of

Europe; in particular Germany, the Netherlands and the UK.[33] To a lesser extent, IVDUs in Italy and Spain also played a role.[34]

The common goal across Europe was to control the spread of infection whether by coercion or autonomy. Coercion, however, is likely to be counterproductive by driving those most at risk underground, and infringing their rights to treatment. Autonomy and privacy on the other hand are more likely to encourage the desired behavioural change.[35]

Legality of HIV testing, detention and compulsory treatment

The European Court of Justice decreed that HIV testing had to be with the patient's specific consent in order to uphold the patient's rights to privacy under European Community Law.[36] Again, the underpinning belief was that the possibility of deception would result in people who were infected or at risk of becoming infected from seeking appropriate medical management.[37] Likewise compulsory testing, detention and isolation would be an infringement of the liberty of the affected persons.[38]

At the time that these policies and laws were decreed there was no vaccine and no cure for AIDS. With the development of Highly Active Anti-Retroviral Therapy (HAART), which involves taking a variable combination of drugs, there has been a dramatic reduction in the viral load rendering the person less infectious to others.[39] This treatment delays the onset of AIDS and therefore overall mortality.[40] The use of anti-retroviral therapy in pregnant women has also reduced perinatal transmission. These advances have led to a reduction in the financial burden to the various health systems and HIV/AIDS has been downgraded from a 'fatal disease' to a 'chronic condition'. As a result AIDS no longer constitutes a state of emergency in Europe. This has helped to reduce the stigmatisation of the infection and consequently the need for specific consent for HIV testing has had to be re-addressed. It could be argued that testing without consent is justifiable (both legally and ethically) in the context of the patient's best interests (e.g. where a person lacks capacity, whether through mental illness/disability or in the unconscious patient). Whether this applies to testing for the benefit of others not yet infected remains undecided.

The argument for compulsory testing must also be re-evaluated since the sooner HAART is commenced the more likely it is to benefit the patient in terms of quality and quantity of life.[41] With the advent of HAART, AIDS is no longer classified as a fatal disease, so there is less risk of stigmatisation with compulsory testing.

While mass screening for HIV is considered inappropriate, some countries have implemented selective testing of certain high-risk populations.

In the UK and France it is policy to offer all pregnant women HIV tests at antenatal clinics. In America pregnant women who are also IVDUs have been targeted for compulsory testing in order to protect the foetus.[42,43]

THE LEGAL FRAMEWORK IN THE UK

The only specific piece of legislation in the UK pertaining to HIV – The AIDS (Control) Act came into effect on 15th May 1987. The three original main aims of the act are as follows:

1. To understand the epidemic in the UK
2. To gather information about what the health authorities and local authorities are doing to monitor the infection in order to learn from best practise
3. To help focus at both national and local levels.

Annual reports are made to the Regional Health Authority and the Secretary of State by the District Health Authority by:

- Each regional office in England of the DoH's NHS Management Executive; these offices replaced Regional Health Authorities in England
- Each District Health Authority in Wales
- Each Health Board in Scotland.

Section 23 of the Act prevents the sale, supply or administration of any equipment or reagents to detect HIV antibodies (test kits) in centres without medical supervision and no certainty of pre- and post-test counselling.

With the development of effective treatment, new challenges arose to ensure that health services were able to target and provide treatment to the appropriate people. In 1999 the All-Party Parliamentary Group on AIDS decided to introduce changes to make the workings of the 1987 Act more relevant. Under the initial Act where they were less than 10 cases in a given area, they were reported as an asterisk for fear of low-prevalence areas being identified. It was felt that since the climate had changed and it was possible to maintain confidentiality these areas should be reported.

Secondly, the data needed to include people resident in a health authority area as well as those merely diagnosed or appearing for services in that area to provide a more comprehensive picture and enable a more accurate basis for planning and monitoring prevention work and social service work. They also wanted to ensure that Government money was being spent effectively on those most at risk of acquiring HIV.

They suggested that the Act be amended to require the reports to show total expenditure on recognised target groups.

Other relevant legislation includes the Public Health (Control of Disease) Act 1984 and the Public Health (Infectious Diseases) Regulations, 1985 and1988, which makes certain diseases notifiable. Hepatitis B, C and D are included in this, but not HIV. However, the Public Health (Infectious Disease) Regulations 1985/1988 allow Sections 35 (medical examination), 37 (removal to hospital), 38 (detention in hospital), 43 (restrictions on removal of the body of person dying in hospital) and 44 (isolation of the body of a person dying outside hospital) to apply.

A single Justice of the Peace (acting *ex parte* if necessary) can activate Sections 35, 37 and 38. Compulsory medical examination can only be ordered if the magistrate is satisfied that there is reason to believe that a person is suffering from a notifiable disease. For this to occur, the magistrate must receive a written certificate (in the form set out in schedule 2 of the 1988 regulations, or a 'similar form substantially to the like effect') confirming this from a medical practitioner nominated by the local authority.

The 1985 Regulations were superseded by the 1988 Regulations and removed the words '*or is carrying an organism capable of causing it*'. The order can only be made if it is in the interests of the patient, the family or the public and must have the consent of the registered medical practitioner treating the patient. Section 35 orders can be supplemented by orders under Section 61 of the 1985 Regulations allowing magistrates to issue warrants to support the entry, if necessary by force, of an authorised officer. Wilful neglect or refusal to obey, or obstruction of the Regulations may be punishable by a fine under Section 15.

Section 37 allows a local authority to apply to a magistrate to remove an AIDS patient to hospital. The 1988 Public Health (Infectious Diseases) Regulations 1988 has modified Section 38(1) of the original Act as applied to AIDS. This modification allows a Justice of the Peace (acting *ex parte* if deemed necessary), following the application of any local authority, to make an order for the detention in hospital of an inmate of that hospital suffering from AIDS. This can only be carried out if the Justice of the Peace is satisfied that on leaving the hospital the patient would not take proper precautions to prevent the spread of that disease

(a) In their lodging or accommodation, or
(b) In other places in which they may be expected to go if not detained in the hospital.

Compulsory action would only be considered where there is clear evidence of risk. For BBVs this would apply to an individual who had uncontrollable bleeding. This section of the Act may also apply to other notifiable diseases, e.g. uncontrolled infective diarrhoea, and drug-resistant pulmonary or disseminated tuberculosis. The individual has the right to appeal against Sections 35, 37 and 38 by applying to the Crown Court. Judicial review is also available to challenge procedural errors or matters of jurisdiction.

On September 14th 1985, magistrates in Manchester, UK, ordered that a 25-year old man with AIDS be detained for 3 weeks in Monsall Hospital under Section 38. The City Council Medical Officer for Environmental Health said that the patient was 'bleeding copiously and trying to discharge himself'. At the Crown Court appeal, Mr. Justice Russell allowed the man to be released, as he was advised by Counsel for the City that the man's condition had improved substantially and continued detention was no longer sought. Mr Russell added that the original order was 'proper in view of the medical evidence'. As the man was now willing to stay in hospital, the appeal was uncontested and no case law was created.[44]

Cadavers may also pose infection hazards to people who handle them. The use of appropriate protective clothing and the observance of the Control of Substances Hazardous to Health Regulations (COSHH) regulations will protect anyone handling cadavers from acquiring an infectious disease. Bodies infected with hepatitis B, C or D must be bagged, but cannot be embalmed, or hygienically prepared. (The latter involves cleaning and tidying of the body before viewing.) It is also advised that bodies of those dying with HIV/AIDS should be bagged, but is not an absolute requirement. However, neither embalming nor hygienic preparation are allowed.[45] HIV may survive for days after death in tissues preserved under laboratory conditions.[46]

If a person dies of AIDS in hospital, a 'proper officer of the local authority' can certify (under Section 43 of the Public Health (Control of Disease) Act 1984) that the body should not be removed except for transfer to a mortuary or for cremation or burial. A 'proper officer' is usually the consultant in Communicable Disease Control. Cremation can only take place provided that the Medical Referee (approved by the Secretary of State for the Home Department) is satisfied that the cause of death has been definitely ascertained. Disregard of a certificate is a criminal offence, punishable by a fine.

HIV is also covered by the National Health Service (Venereal Diseases) Regulations 1974. Under this act health authorities have a duty not to disclose any information capable of identifying an individual examined or treated for a sexually transmitted disease. This confidentiality may only be breached in exceptional circumstances. In 1988, in the case of *X v Y*[47] the court banned a newspaper from using information wrongly extracted from the confidential notes of two medical practitioners with AIDS. It was upheld that public interests were outweighed against loyalty and confidentiality both generally and in relation to AIDS patients' hospital records.[48]

The risk from infected blood products and the law

In October 1985, following the development of reliable tests for HIV, Factor VIII NHS concentrates were heat-treated to render them safe.

In November 1987, the Government set up a £10 million trust fund for affected haemophiliacs and their families, to make *ex gratia* payments (an average of £8500 per family) and not as compensation. In July 1989, the Lord Chief Justice assigned to Mr Justice Ognall the cases of several patients with haemophilia and HIV infection and their families who were suing, or proposed to sue the Government and Health Authorities, with the intention of co-ordination along the lines of the 'Opren' litigation.[49] On 11 December 1990, an out of court settlement was made by the DoH of £42 million for 1217 haemophiliacs known to be infected with AIDS.

Following the identification of HCV in 1989 and the availability of a reliable test in 1991, the National Blood Authority started screening donations. On 11 January 1995, the DoH announced that 3000 former hospital patients (survivors of an original total of more than 6000) who had received blood transfusions prior to September 1991 were being contacted, because treatment was now available. The Government rejected claims for compensation for haemophiliacs who had contracted hepatitis C through contaminated blood products on 30th January of the same year.

UK CASE LAW

In the first half of 1993 at least 14 injecting drug users in Glenochil Prison became infected with HIV by needle sharing.[50] In June 1993 Mr Stephen Kelly participated in the infection control exercise having realised that he was at risk. He accepted HIV counselling and testing from an external counsellor who told him of his diagnosis and gave him post-test counselling. Subsequent molecular studies showed that 13 of the 14 had the same strain of virus. These studies also showed that Mr Kelly (one of the 13) had passed the same strain via unprotected vaginal and anal intercourse to Miss Anne Craig in early 1994 – after he had been diagnosed with HIV and had received post-test counselling. Mr Kelly was later sentenced to 5 years imprisonment for 'culpably and recklessly transmitting HIV infection' to Ms Craig. At the time of his relationship with Ms Craig, it was not known that receptive anal intercourse posed a 20 times greater risk of transmitting HIV than by vaginal sex.[51] Neither was it known that the risk was 200 times greater if intercourse occurred during the first 3 months of HIV infection.[52] Therefore, he was unaware of this information. Although Ms Craig knew of Mr Kelly's drug-injecting history and that he had been in prison he had not informed her that he was HIV positive. This fact played a major part in the trial and the sentence he received. As a result of the Kelly verdict, it is now a crime under Scottish law for someone who knows they are HIV positive and conceals the knowledge to have unprotected sexual contact with another person and to transmit infection. The same rule does not apply to someone who has not been tested and is therefore unaware of their infection.

The judgement also raises other doubts as to which behaviours are criminal. Bird and Leigh Brown[53] posed the following questions:

- Is it a crime to for someone who conceals their HIV infection to have unprotected intercourse if HIV transmission does not occur?
- Could someone who conceals their HIV infection be prosecuted if they have protected intercourse that results in HIV transmission, because, for example, a condom breaks?

They suggest that both could constitute a crime if analogies are made with other crimes against the person, as demonstrated by the Cuerrier judgement in Canada. The latter has made HIV disclosure to sexual partners obligatory, even if condoms are always used[54]. The full impact of the Glenochil judgement under Scottish law has yet to be determined. Continued and increased surveillance is needed to see whether fewer at-risk people present for HIV testing, for fear of prosecution. If this happens then people who have HIV infection and are not diagnosed will not receive HAART. It may also lead to an increase in other people becoming infected whether through sexual contact or sharing drug paraphernalia.

The judgement may also impact on HIV counsellors if they are found to be negligent in informing their clients of the change in the law in Scotland. However, it still remains the responsibility of the infected person to inform contacts deemed at risk providing that they have been appropriately counselled. It could also affect the numbers of people willing to contribute samples for molecular studies, since in the case of *R v Kelly* the police used a warrant to access unnamed molecular research data and made the information forensic evidence.

UK GUIDANCE TO HCWs

Health Authorities, NHS and Primary Care Trusts have a duty to protect HCWs from the occupational acquisition of BBVs and from infected HCWs from infecting patients. Under the Health Service Circular produced by the DoH and the Public Health Laboratory Service in 1998,[55] each employer is responsible for drawing up a policy on the management of blood exposure incidents for both staff and patients. Independent contractors in the General Medical and Dental Services should also ensure that they have similar arrangements in place.

The risk to HCWs of acquiring infection from a patient is greater than converse. To June 1999 a total of 102 definitive cases of HIV-seroconversion following a specific occupational exposure have been reported worldwide.

USA	55
Europe (including UK)	35
Rest of World	12
Total	102

A further 217 possible occupationally acquired infections (with no presumed other risk factors have been reported. However, the occupational risk depends on the population prevalence of HIV and the safety of working conditions. 92% of all occupationally acquired infections have been reported from countries with good surveillance systems, the majority of which have low HIV prevalence. Only 5% of cases have come from African countries, with none from the Indian Subcontinent or South East Asia. These countries have a high prevalence of HIV with poor monitoring systems.

In the UK safe working practices under the Health and Safety at Work Act 1974, the Environmental Protection Act (1990) and the COSHH (1994) together with the DoH guidelines have helped to reduce the likelihood of such an incident occurring. The latter include:

- Establishing guidelines for managing occupational exposures and designating a specific person/team to deal with such incidents (see specific sections)
- The implementation of hepatitis B vaccination of HCWs under the 1993 HSG[56]

- The introduction of Post Exposure Prophylaxis following potential exposure to HIV[57,58]
- Early monitoring for hepatitis C and where appropriate the administration of Ribavirin and Interferon.[59]

Equally all HCWs have an ethical and legal duty to protect the patients under their care. They should never knowingly place a patient at risk. The General Medical Council's guidance Good Medical Practice and Serious Communicable Diseases upholds this view. It states that

> doctors who have a serious communicable disease and continue in their professional practise must have appropriate medical supervision and should not rely upon their own assessments of the risks they pose to patients.

The DoH has also issued guidelines relevant to the specific BBVs. These guidelines are regularly reviewed and updated to maintain and minimise the risk of such transmissions. They apply to all HCWs who carry out Exposure Prone Procedures (EPP that is there is a risk that injury to the HCW could result in their blood contaminating a patient's open tissues. EPPs occur mainly in surgery (including some minor surgery carried out by General Physicians, GPs), obstetrics and gynaecology, dentistry and midwifery. A full list is contained in Guidance on the management of HIV/AIDS infected healthcare workers and patient notification. (Health Service Circular 1998/226)). HCWs include those who work in the NHS; ambulance staff; independent contractors such as dental and medical practitioners (and relevant staff); independent midwives; students; podiatrists; locums and agency staff; and visiting HCWs. The National Minimum Standards for Independent Health Care (DoH 2002) require workers in the independent health sector to comply with D0H guidelines if they are infected with a BBV.

GENERAL PRINCIPLES APPLYING TO BBVs

- HCWs who are infected with any of these viruses and could potentially infect a patient are now restricted in their working practise.
- The Association of NHS Occupational Physicians (ANHOPs) and the Association of NHS Occupational Health Nurse Advisors (ANHONA) have agreed on the standards required for occupational health data recording.
- Laboratory tests required for clearance for performing EPPS can only be derived from an 'identified validated sample' (IVS) before they are recorded in occupational health records.

Criteria for an IVS

- HCW must show proof of identity with a photograph when the sample is taken
- The sample should be taken in the Occupational Health Department (OHD) or by another specifically designated person
- HCWs should not provide their own samples
- Samples must be transported to the laboratory in the usual manner and *not* by the HCW
- Laboratory results received by the OHD should be checked to ensure that the sample was sent by the OHD

Only accredited laboratories can carry out the necessary tests and such laboratories must participate in appropriate external quality assurance schemes.

- The HCW has the same right to confidentiality as accorded to a patient. However, health clearance certificates issued by OHDs must make it clear whether the employee has been cleared to perform EPPs.
- The specific reason for non-clearance should not normally be disclosed without the consent from the HCW.
- However, where patients are, or have been at risk, it may be necessary in the public interest for the 'employer' to receive confidential information. This decision will be made on a case-by-case basis using three risk assessment criteria.
  - Evidence of possible HIV transmission
  - The nature and history of the infected healthcare worker's clinical practise
  - Other relevant considerations (e.g. evidence of poor clinical practise in relation to infection control or physical/mental impairment as a result of symptomatic HIV disease.
- Other HCWs have a duty to report if they know or have good reason to believe that an infected HCW has not complied with the DoH guidance or followed advice to modify their practise.
- This report should be made to an appropriate person (e.g. a consultant Occupational Health Physician, Trust medical director or director of public health).
- Such HCWs may wish to seek guidance from their regulatory and professional bodies before disclosing this information.

- HCWs who already know they are infected or are about to undertake training that involves EPPs and fail to comply with the DoH guidelines (e.g. refusing to have the relevant tests) must no longer perform EPPs nor be allowed to start training.
- Patient notification after a potential exposure from an infected HCW should be assessed on a case-by-case basis. Directors of Public Health of Primary Care Trusts or Consultants in Communicable Disease Control are responsible for deciding whether patient notification is necessary. The UK Advisory Panel for Health Care Workers Infected with Blood-borne Viruses (UKAP) are also available to give advice.[59–61]

SPECIFIC GUIDELINES

Hepatitis B

Health Service Guidelines were first issued in 1993[56] and were updated in 1996 and 2000.[61]

HCWs infected with hepatitis B must undergo a series of tests to assess the degree of risk they pose to their patients. The results of these tests may restrict areas of practice. Those who are hepatitis B surface antigen (HBsAg) and e antigen positive (HbeAg) are not allowed to perform EPPs. Since there have been several incidents where HbeAg negative HCWs have transmitted hepatitis B to patients during EPPs, any HbeAg negative HCW performing EPPs must undergo a further test to measure viral load. Only two laboratories have been designated to perform this test:

- The Public Health Laboratory, Heartlands Hospital, Birmingham
- The Regional Virus Laboratory, Gartnavel General Hospital, Glasgow

New guidance states that anyone with a viral load $>10^3$ genome equivalents/ml are no longer allowed to perform EPPs. Those with viral loads below 10^3 genome equivalents may continue to perform EPPs, but must be reassessed annually as viral loads may fluctuate.[61]

The Advisory Group on Hepatitis (AGH) has recommended that hepatitis B infected HCWs should not continue to perform EPPs while on interferon or other antiviral therapy. Those who have received treatment will only be considered as to their suitability for unrestricted working practise if they can show that their viral load does not exceed the recommended level 1 year after therapy is completed. If they are eligible, then they would still be subjected to an annual review.

Hepatitis C

The first report of an HCV-infected surgeon transmitting virus to a single patient occurred in 1994[62] and in 1995 the AGH recommended that hepatitis C infected HCWs should no longer perform EPPs.[63] Since then there have been four further incidents in the UK involving 14 patients. As a result the AGH have made further recommendations to minimise patient risk. These have been incorporated into Health Service Circular 2002–2010.[59]

HCV testing is currently recommended for the following groups. It does not include all staff or medical students at the present time, but this is under review.

- HCW who already know they have been infected with HCV and who perform EPPs should be tested for HCV RNA. If they are found to be RNA positive they cannot continue to perform EPPs.
- HCWs who are intending to undertake a career that involves the performance of EPPs should be tested for HCV antibodies prior to commencement of training. If they are antibody positive then HCV RNA tests will be performed. They will be restricted from training if they are RNA positive. This group includes junior doctors entering all surgical specialities (including A&E) prior to their first SHO post, GP trainees intending to perform minor surgery, ambulance staff, podiatrists, theatre and A&E nurses, prospective midwifery students and dental students.
- HCWs who perform EPPs and believe they may have been exposed to HCV should seek advice as soon as possible (e.g. from an occupational health physician).
- HCWs who have responded successfully to anti-viral therapy (i.e. remain HCV RNA negative 6 months after the end of treatment) may resume work or start training. Further checks should be carried out 6 months later to ensure they are still RNA-negative.
- Qualitative testing for HCV RNA must be carried out by accredited laboratories. The assays used should have a minimum sensitivity of 50 IU/ml. Two samples are taken a week apart.

HIV

There have only been two reports worldwide of possible HIV transmission from a healthcare worker performing an EPPs: a French orthopaedic surgeon[64] and a Florida dentist.[65] The route of transmission was only clearly demonstrated in the former case. All other retrospective studies carried out have failed to show transmission from an infected healthcare worker to a patient. This is supported by data collected in the UK between 1998 and 2001. Twenty-two notification exercises were carried out testing 7000 patients, but no evidence of HIV transmission was found.

As with the other BBVs, HCWs who are HIV positive must not perform EPPs. Neither should they carry out EPPs if they are awaiting test results. All HCWs should be offered an HIV antibody test if they consider that they might have been exposed to HIV through the following routes:

- Unprotected sexual intercourse between men
- Sharing injecting equipment while misusing drugs
- Unprotected heterosexual intercourse in, or with a person, exposed in a country where heterosexual HIV transmission is common
- Involvement in invasive medical, surgical, dental or midwifery procedures in parts of the world where infection control precautions might have been inadequate, or with populations with a high prevalence of HIV
- Significant occupational exposure to HIV infected material in any circumstances
- Engaged in unprotected sexual intercourse with someone in any of the above categories.

HIV infected HCWs applying for new posts should complete health questionnaires honestly. Any healthcare worker who is about to embark on a career that involves EPPs must now be tested prior to starting training.[66,67] A positive test is only considered relevant if the individual intends to perform EPPs. However, in accordance with good practice, any healthcare worker found to be HIV positive should remain under medical and occupational health supervision.

Under The Disability Discrimination Act 1995 it is unlawful to discriminate against disabled persons including those with HIV infection or AIDS in any area of employment (even HCWs performing EPPs). However, the employer has a duty to find an alternative post, if available. Asymptomatic HIV infection does not currently apply to this legislation.

UK LEGISLATION UNDER REVIEW

Section 9A of the Misuse of Drugs Act 1971 currently makes it an offence for a person to supply any article – other than needles and syringes – in cases where the supplier believes that it may be used to administer an unlawful drug. Needles and syringes were not included in order to reduce the risk of BBVs. However, evidence arose to suggest that other items of drug paraphernalia also posed a risk and so the Advisory Council on the Misuse of Drugs (ACMD) was asked to consider other items. Their findings indicated that certain other items constituted a valid risk.

As a result of their investigation the government have proposed that the supply of the following articles of paraphernalia be made lawful in order to further reduce the risk of harm to drug users:[68]

- Sterile water ampoules
- Swabs
- Spoons
- Bowls
- Citric acid

The following items are not included as there was either insufficient evidence to substantiate a risk, or there was evidence that it could encourage drug-injecting behaviour:

- Tourniquets
- Filters
- Cigarette papers

The ACMD recommended that citric acid should only be supplied by pharmacists and others who have had appropriate training on its effects and the quantities to be used, as its use could lead to burns at injection sites and other medical complications.

Water ampoules are currently classified as a 'Prescription Only Medicine' (POM) under the medicines legislation and can therefore only be supplied by a pharmacist with a doctor's prescription. The ACMD felt it was necessary to re-examine the POMs (Human Use) Order 1997, to allow water ampoules to be supplied by other healthcare professionals working in drug treatment services.

The Home Secretary proposes to make the amendments through secondary legislation, using the powers under Sections 22(a) and 31 of the Misuse of Drugs act 1971. These amending regulations would countermand the Section 9A provisions in certain circumstances to make it lawful for authorised persons to supply certain articles of paraphernalia. The proposals would facilitate the supply of such articles to drug misusers by NHS Specialist Drug Units, pharmacists and by charities and voluntary organisations that run drug agencies. There has been no special funding allocated for this, so the various agencies would have to be able to supply the items out of their existing budgets.

The proposed changes to the misuse of drug legislation would have an effect in England, Wales and Scotland. However, the existence of common law crimes in Scotland – in particular the crime of reckless conduct – means that it is not possible to say that the supply of drugs paraphernalia could never amount to a criminal offence. However, the proposals have been welcomed by the Scottish Executive, who intends to review existing guidance on needle-exchange systems to take account of the supply of drugs paraphernalia. The Lord Advocate would not authorise prosecution of any doctor/staff participating in such schemes as long as they have adhered to the approved arrangements. Northern Ireland has its own separate misuse of drug regulations. Amendments for Northern Ireland could be made using the powers under Sections 22(a), 30(4) and 31 or the MDA 1971.

The legislative changes are due to be implemented in 2003 subject to further comments and advice. Only the listed items would be considered lawful and the specified suppliers would no longer be considered as committing an offence. However, agencies that supply 'drug paraphernalia kits' incorporating filters, tourniquets and/or cigarette papers, would still be liable to prosecution.

SUMMARY

By the continued and careful monitoring of the prevalence of BBVs a clearer picture will emerge of the impact of the viruses on the world. Each country must strive to improve health education and make treatments available. They must also try to avoid stigmatisation that would discourage reporting of infections to the relevant bodies, as was seen with the initial 'knee-jerk' responses that followed the discovery of HIV. For example, in industrialised countries, insurance companies penalised anyone undergoing a test for HIV antibodies regardless of the test outcome. Fortunately this is no longer the case.

Any future changes in legislation (whether at an international or national level) must be made with care in order to preserve the rights of the individual, while protecting others who could be placed at risk. The laws need to be clear to avoid the confusion and contentious issues that have previously arisen. For example, whether someone is culpable in law of knowingly infecting another person still remains to be resolved depending on the country (and within the USA – the State) of origin.

There is no doubt, that the law will continue to play a role in developing policies. But it should not be at the expense of those who are most at risk of acquiring infection from obtaining the appropriate treatment.

REFERENCES AND FURTHER READING

1. Centers for Disease Control of Prevention, Atlanta, Georgia. Division of Viral Hepatitis. National Center for Infectious Diseases. Hepatitis D slide set – updated May 16th 2003.
2. Hepatitis D Virus. Howard J Worman, 1995, 2003. Hepatitiscentral.com
3. Hepatitis D. Sean Lacey, Dept of Medicine, Case Western Reserve University. Last update September 6th 2001.
4. CDC, Atlanta 1981, MMWR 30: 250. Pneumocystis pneumonia – Los Angeles. CDC, Atlanta.
5. 1981, MMWR 30: 305. Kaposi's Sarcoma and Pneumocystis Pneumonia among Homosexual men – New York City and California.
6. Choi KH, Liu M, Guo Y et al. Emerging HIV-1 epidemic in China in men who have sex with men. *Lancet* 2003, 361 9375: 2125–6.
7. The UN Theme Group on HIV/AIDS in China. HIV/AIDS: China's titanic peril, 2001 update of the AIDS situation and needs assessment report. Geneva, Switzerland: UNAIDS, 2002.
8. Beach M. China responds to increasing HIV/AIDS burden and holds landmark meeting. *Lancet* 2001, 358: 1792.
9. Loveday C, Pomeroy L, Weller IVD *et al.* Human immunodeficiency viruses in patients attending a sexually transmitted disease clinic in London, 1982–1987. *Brit. Med. J.* 1989, 298: 419–421.
10. Paget W, Zwahlen M, Eichmann A, Swiss Network of DP. Voluntary confidential HIV testing of STD patients in Switzerland, 1990–1995; HIV test refusers cause different biases on HIV prevalence in heterosexuals and homo/bisexuals. *Genitourin Med.* 1997, 43: 444–447.
11. Heptonstall J, Gill ON. The legal and ethical basis for unlinked anonymous HIV testing. *Commun. Dis. Rep.* 1989, 48: 3–6.
12. AIDS/HIV Quarterly Surveillance Tables. Cumulative data to end December 2002. Public Health Laboratory Surveillance AIDS centre (HIV/STI Division) CDSC and the Scottish Centre for Infection and Environmental Health, No. 57: 02/4. February, 2003.
13. European Collaborative Study. Risk factors for mother-to-child transmission of HIV-1. *Lancet* 1992, 339: 1007–1012.
14. International Perinatal HIV group. Mode of vertical transmission of HIV-1. A metanalysis of fifteen prospective cohort studies. *New Eng. J. Med.* 1999, 340: 977–987.
15. Duong T, Ades A, Gibbs DM, *et al.* Vertical transmission rate for HIV in the British Isles estimated on Surveillance data. *Brit. Med. J.* 1999, 319: 1227–1229.
16. National Institutes of Allergy and Infectious Diseases. National Institutes of Health, Bethesda, MD, USA. Mother-to-Infant HIV Transmission Rate Less Than 2 Percent in Phase III Perinatal Trial. Press Release. July 2002.
17. Occupational transmission of HIV. Summary of Published reports. Data to end of June 1999. Published December 1999. PHLS AIDS and STD Centre at CDSC.
18. Alter MJ. The epidemiology of acute and chronic hepatitis C. *Clin. Liv. Dis.* 1997, 1: 559–562.

19. Frank C *et al.* The role of the parenteral antischistosomal therapy in the spread of hepatitis C virus in Egypt. *Lancet* 2000, 355: 887–891.

20. Chronic Hepatitis C: Disease Management. NIH publication No. 03-4230. February 2003.

21. Hope VD, Judd A, Hickman M, Lamagni T, Hunter G, *et al.* Prevalence of hepatitis C among injection drug users in England and Wales: is harm reduction working? *Am. J. Public Health* 2001, 91(1): 38–42.

22. Hepatitis C Strategy for England. Implementing Getting Ahead of the Curve: A Strategy for combating Infectious Diseases. Department of Health 14/8/2002.

23. M.E. Ramsay *et al.* Laboratory surveillance of hepatitis C virus infection in England and Wales: 1992 to 1996. *Commun. Dis. Public Health*, 1(2), June 1998. pp. 89–94.

24. Hamblin J. The Role of the Law in HIV and AIDS Policy. *HIV Development Programme* 1991, Issues paper No. 11.

25. Anonymous: St. Valentine's Revenge. *Lancet* 1991, 337: 548.

26. Godwin J, Hamblin J, Patterson D. *Australian HIV/AIDS Legal Guide*. Sydney: The Federation Press, 1991, pp. 182.

27. Gostin LO. The AIDS Litigation Project: a national review of court and human rights commission decisions. Part II: Discrimination, *JAMA* 1990, 263: 2086–2093.

28. Hamblin J, Somerville MA. Surveillance and reporting of HIV infection and AIDS in Canada: ethics and law. *Univ. Toronto Law J.* 1991, 41: 224–246.

29. Rule of law – HIV/AIDS and human rights; international guidelines. Geneva: UNAIDS and Office of the High Commissioner for Human Rights, 1998 (HR/PUB/98/1).

30. Office of the United Nations High Commission for Human Rights and the joint United Nations Programme on HIV/AIDS. *Third international consultation of HIV/AIDS and human rights.* Geneva: OHCHR and UNAIDS, 2002.

31. Hendriksson B, Yetterberg H. Sweden: the power of moral (istic) left. In Kirp DL, Bayer R, (eds), *AIDS In the Industrialized Democracies: Passions, Politics, Policies* (pp. 315–338). Camden NJ: Rutgers International Press, 1992.

32. Hofmann J. Verfassungs-und verwaltungreschtliche Probleme der Virus-Erkrankung AIDS unter besonderer Berucksichtigung des bayerischen Massnahmenkatalogs. *Neue Juritische Wochenschrift* 1988, 41: 1486–1494.

33. Berridge V. *AIDS in the UK: The Making of Policy*, 1981–1994. Oxford: Oxford University Press, 1996.

34. Moss D. AIDS in Italy: Emergence in slow motion. In Misztal BA and Moss D (eds), *Action on AIDS: National Policies in Comparative Perspective* (pp. 135–166). Westport CT: Greenwood Press, 1990.

35. Buchanan D. The law and HIV transmission: help or hindrance? *Venereology* 1999, 12: 57–66.

36. *X v Commission of the European Communities*, 1994, European Court Reports 1-4737 (ECJ).

37. Wright M. Testing for HIV and consent: law and public policy. *Med. Law Inter.* 1994, 1: 221–239.

38. Acheson ED. AIDS: A challenge for the public health. *Lancet* 1988, 1: (8482), 662–666.

39. Royce RA, Sena A, Cates W, Cohen MS. Sexual transmission of HIV: Current concepts. *New Eng. J. Med.* 1997, 336: 1072.

40. Cohn JA. Recent advances: HIV infection I. *BMJ* 1997, 314: 487–491.

41. Ho DD. Time to hit HIV, early and hard. *New Eng. J. Med.* 1995, 333: 450–451.

42. McGovern T. Mandatory HIV testing and treating child-bearing women: An unnatural, illegal and unsound approach. *Columbia Human Rights Rev.* 1997, 28: 469–499.

43. Halem SC. At what cost? – an argument against mandatory AZT treatment of HIV-positive women. *Harvard Civil Rights – Civil Liberties Rev.* 1997, 32: 491–544.

44. BMJ Legal Correspondent. Detaining patients with AIDS. *BMJ* 1985, 291: 1102.

45. Healing TD, Hoffman PN, Young SEJ. Communicable Disease Report. The infection hazards of human cadavers. *CDR Rev.* 1995, 5 No. 5.

46. Ball J, Desselberger U, Whitwell H. Long-lasting viability of HIV after patient's death. *Lancet* 1991, 338: 63.

47. *X (Health Authority) v Y*, 1988, 2 All ER 648.

48. Dyer C. Doctors with AIDS and the 'News of the World'. *Brit. Med. J.* 1987, 295: 1102.

49. *Nash v Eli Lilly*, 1991, 2 Med LR 169.

50. Christie B. HIV outbreak investigated in Scottish Jail. *Brit. Med. J.* 1993, 307: 151–152.

51. Fielding KL, Brettle RP, Gore SM, O'Brien F, Wyld R, Robertson JR, *et al*. Heterosexual transmission of HIV analysed by generalized estimating equations. *Stat. Med.* 1995, 14: 1365–1378.

52. Leynaert B, Downs AM, de Vincenzi I. European Study Group on Heterosexual Transmission of HIV. *Heterosexual transmission of human immunodeficiency virus. Variability of infectivity throughout the course of infection. Am. J. Epidemiol.* 1998, 148: 88–96.

53. Bird SM, Leigh Brown AJ. Criminalisation of HIV transmission: implications for public health in Scotland. *Brit. Med. J.* 2001, 323: 1174–1177.

54. Elliott R. Supreme Court rules in R *v* Cuerrier. *Canadian HIV/AIDS Policy and Law Newsletter* 1999, 4(2/3): 16–23.

55. Guidance for Clinical Health Care Workers: Protection against infection with blood-borne viruses. Recommendations of the Expert Advisory Group on AIDS and the Advisory Group on Hepatitis. Health Service Circular (HSC 1998/063).

56. Protecting healthcare workers and patients from hepatitis B: recommendations of the Advisory Group on Hepatitis. Department of Health, HSC 1993/(93)/40.

57. Guidance on post-exposure prophylaxis for health care workers occupationally exposed to HIV. Department of Health PL/CO (97) 1.

58. HIV Post-Exposure Prophylaxis: Guidance from the UK Chief Medical Officer's Expert Advisory Group on AIDS. July 2000.

59. DOH guidelines Health Service Circular HSC 2002/010. Hepatitis C infected health care workers. (14 August 2002). See http://www.doh.gov.uk/hepatitisc.

60. HIV Infected Health Care Workers. Implementing 'Getting Ahead of the Curve' action on blood-borne viruses. (A Consultation Paper on Management and Patient Notification) DOH 2002.

61. Hepatitis B infected Health Care Workers. Guidance on implementation of Health Service Circular 2000 (020). Published June 2000.

62. Duckworth GJ, Heptonstall J, *et al.* Transmission of hepatitis C virus from a surgeon to a patient. *Commun. Dis. Public Health* 1999, 2: 188–192.

63. CDSC. Hepatitis C virus transmission from health care worker to patient. *Commun. Dis. Rep. CDR Wkly* 1995, 5: 121.

64. Lot F, Séguier J-C, Fégueux S, Astagneau P, Simon P, Aggoune M, *et al.* Probable transmission of HIV from an orthopaedic surgeon to a patient in France. *Ann. Intern. Med.* 1999, 130: 1–6.

65. Ciesielski C, Marianos D, Ou C-Y, Dunbaugh R, Witte J, Berkelman R, *et al.* Transmission of human immunodeficiency virus in a dental practice. *Ann. Intern. Med.* 1992, 116: 798–805.

66. Guidance on the management of AIDS/HIV infected health care workers and patient notification. Health Service Circular HSC 1998/226.

67. HIV Infected Health Care Worker. Implementing 'Getting Ahead of the Curve': action on blood-borne viruses. DOH Draft Guidance 2002.

68. Proposals to make lawful the supply of specific items of drug paraphernalia to drug users. (Issued in a letter from the Organised Crime and Drugs International Group, November 2002.)

20

Healthcare professionals in court – professional and expert witnesses

Stephen Robinson

INTRODUCTION

This chapter addresses issues relevant for preparing and giving evidence. Though the title mentions court the main principles involved apply wherever that person gives evidence. The range is quite large and includes, criminal courts, civil courts, death investigation (Coroners Courts in England and Wales and Fatal Accident Inquiries in Scotland for example), family courts, child protection conferences, employment and discipline tribunals.

The term 'court' will be used but the same principles apply whatever the form of the tribunal. The healthcare professional may be involved in court in two ways, as a professional witness to fact or as an expert witness where the role may be to express opinions on the role of others. There are two stages to any evidence giving process, the first is the preparation of a written document, the second is the attendance at the court to give live testimony.

A report is a written way of transferring information between professionals within the same discipline or across discipline boundaries. It also allows the information involved to be accessed at a later date and on numerous occasions without the author being present.

A statement in this context is viewed as a specialised format of a report. In medico-legal matters the content should be same whether the specialised format is used or not. The content and thrust of a report may vary slightly depending on its purpose. For example a report for a child protection case may have a different emphasis than the statement produced if criminal charges are an issue.

A report prepared for a civil case has specific requirements which will be dealt with below. The statement in criminal matters is a way of providing evidence which is as valid as evidence had been given live. It is for that reason that a declaration is signed when constructing a statement in England and Wales. Any dishonesty in a signed statement is the same as perjury when giving live testimony. Slightly different formats are used in Scotland, Northern Ireland, The Channel Islands and the Isle of Man, but should the statement be needed for cross jurisdiction purposes, for example if a suspect is arrested away from the alleged crime scene, then the appropriate format would be provided if necessary. In England and Wales this form of statement is often referred to as a 'Section 9' statement because of the statutory instrument which allowed evidence to be given in that way. The statement carries a declaration thus:

> This statement (consisting of ... pages each signed by me), is true to the best of my knowledge and belief and I make it knowing that, if it is tendered in evidence, I shall be liable to prosecution if I have wilfully stated in it anything which I know to be false or do not believe to be true.

Though the declaration does not indicate as such, an omission could be just as improper as an invalid piece of information which is included. It must always be remembered that the healthcare professional has an overriding duty to the court. This does not mean that the individual has no duty to the patient. But whether the person, who is the subject of the report, is a patient of the professional at the time or not once called upon to give evidence then there is a prime duty to be totally honest to the court no matter whether this is to the individual patients' advantage or not. Of course if the individual is or has been a patient of the healthcare professional then appropriate consent should be obtained from the patient and/or parent in the case of a minor before providing any information to the court. In the UK, except in some very specific areas, there is no absolute privilege of even a doctor-patient relationship. Thus it may be that disclosure of information in a report or subsequently by direct evidence can be ordered by a court.

The statement starts with good contemporaneous notes i.e. those notes written at the time of, or very near the time of, examination. Its total factual content should be based on contemporaneous documents and records. Memory can be fickle.

Even if the notes have an omission, which is later included in the statement, it would be better to add an addendum to the original record concerning the additional material and dated and timed to indicate its insertion into the original contemporaneous note.

A statement is made up of a number of parts, including a reprise of the factual information and an opinion. For ease of preparation a statement needs to be broken up into areas.

The statement should wherever possible be typed. Ideally the use of a word processor allows not only an easy way of correcting the presentation during the writing but also of keeping much of the information

About yourself	Name/qualifications/length and depth of experience/post held/posts previously held
About the subject of the report	identification/date, time and duration of examination/place of examination/purpose of examination & consent obtained
History of events	i.e. presenting complaint with relevant history of presenting complaint where applicable to clinical presentation
Examination findings	relevant positive and negative
Investigations performed	including samples taken in a primary forensic examination
Treatment	if any was given (if relevant), including referral to other healthcare resources
Opinion and prognosis	if appropriate

already formatted in place. This is particularly useful if the healthcare professional regularly or frequently prepares such reports. Thus it is possible to have the declaration and all the individual practitioner's own details already set up in the database. The use of paragraphs, indents and outline numbers is perfectly acceptable and often makes for easier reading and understanding.

The statement needs to be carefully prepared during protected time. Writing a statement while being constantly interrupted is likely to lead to errors which will result in frustration at the very best and the potential for a miscarriage of justice at the worst. It should be reviewed closely when completed to ensure typographics errors are corrected, and to ensure that simple errors (e.g. transposition of right for left) are avoided. The contemporaneous notes should be used to construct the statement. If during the writing, omissions or inaccuracies are noticed then the contemporaneous record should be modified in a way which makes it absolutely clear, the circumstances and timing of that modification (e.g. substitution of left for right).

Having completed the standard introduction, then the checklist above can be followed to fill in the details of the individual case. The introductory paragraph should include your name and qualifications. Your qualifications should be typed in full. For example, if a medical practitioner, the term 'ChB' means little to the lay person. But 'Bachelor of Surgery' immediately indicates your standing as a medical professional. Include all relevant qualifications, thus basic medical/nursing/scientific degrees, Royal College qualifications, higher degrees in medicine, law or related sciences and appropriate diplomas should be included. The insertion of qualifications unrelated to the subjects of health and law should be resisted even though they are well earned. The position held should be stated. Your length of service should be stated as should your depth of experience and significant training courses attended. The advantage of this is that the courts will be able to determine how far they may stretch your ability to opine about your findings. In addition it disarms counsel from undermining your credibility during cross-examination, a tactic barristers may wish to use if the facts are not in their favour. In addition the dates, time and place of your contacts with the subject of the report should be declared, including your role at the time of involvement in the case.

The history of the topic in question should be covered including anything relevant to the question in issue. The sources of the history should also be mentioned. For example information gathered from other sources such as a parent should be indicated as having such an origin. Information unreported to you is best dealt with by using the phrase 'I was told by … that …' or 'he told me…'. Court procedure may result in phrases such as this being removed but the decision should be made by the court not by yourself.

The examination or treatment can now be detailed. Including sketches, photographs, graphs, charts or other visual aids can be of great help in illustrating the salient points of the report.

If the examination was primarily a forensic one such as may have been conducted on a complainant in an alleged sexual assault then the sample harvest, if there was one, should be listed, using the references made in your contemporaneous notes. The individual to whom the samples were delivered and the time of delivery should also be recorded in the statement. This is important to complete the 'chain of evidence', linking the sample obtained by the doctor with the scientific analysis.

Any relevant investigations which were performed, such as referral for X-ray, should be mentioned, preferably with the result of the investigation or opinion, if available. An opinion may be offered. There is often much confusion as to whether an opinion can be expressed by a professional witness. There should be no doubt that it is the duty of a professional witness, present as a special witness to fact, to give an opinion on his/her own findings. That opinion however should be limited to the degree of expertise held by the witness. The professional witness must remember that they are not there to represent any particular side and, unless in possession of all the facts can only give a restricted opinion. It is wise to remember not to express an opinion which cannot be substantiated by personal experience, education and publications and which is outside your area of expertise.

The statement is a means of communication. It is of no use to produce a document which can only be understood by another healthcare professional of the same craft. Thus use lay words where the meaning is clear, use a lay word in parenthesis after the proper medical term when the lay word may not be accurate. For example the word 'cut' may be obvious to a lay person but does not differentiate between an incision and laceration, whereas the latter two words are frequently confused even by medical practitioners. Use the correct term for the lesion, for example 'incision' with '(sharp cut)' after it. Try to avoid an unnecessary number of words for the same type of lesion. The word 'bruise' when defined by size will cover any bruise and is simple and straight forward and avoids the accusation of the use of jargon if the more old fashioned words of contusion, ecchymosis or purpura, which themselves can be confusing, are invoked.

Be careful when quoting dimensions to list them correctly i.e. consistency in metric and not confusing mm with cm. As with your qualifications do not use abbreviations, unless the full word has been used in full with the short form being clearly indicated. At that point repeated use of abbreviations would be acceptable.

The clinical record is the foundation of all healthcare practise. Even the possession of an eidetic memory would not allow the record of a medical encounter to be scrutinised by another. No matter how proficient the practitioner, without a professionally prepared contemporaneous record, a weakness exists. Thus it can be considered that a report or statement starts even before a request for one in some cases by the establishment of good quality contemporaneous records whatever the specialism craft of the healthcare professional.

Reference was made earlier to civil court report requirements. Reports for civil cases in England and Wales is now controlled by the Civil Procedure Rules. This also carries a declaration of truth and it is suggested that further information is given by those preparing expert reports.

A good written report may obviate the attendance to give live evidence at court. Even if the professional is called to court to give live evidence this should not be construed as indicating that there is anything amiss with the written report. It may be that further and more detailed information is required, or even that a non-healthcare issue is under scrutiny. For example it may be that the date of any intervention or its duration is being questioned rather than what actually happened or what the health issue was.

However if attending court it is important to remember a number of issues. The most important person in a criminal court is the defendant. It is the duty of anyone giving evidence to be fair and impartial. Any other action is usurping the power of the court as well as being immoral and unethical. Preparation for giving evidence starts with the contemporaneous record. When the court date is imminent ensure a copy of the report and the records used to compile the report are available and in an order which will allow evidence to be given in a professional and controlled manner. Read through the notes before going to court. Seek and find any reference that may have been referred to in the statement. Make certain of the location of the court and double check as to which court is expecting your attendance. Some districts have combined court centres, others may have Crown and Magistrates Courts in buildings separated by some miles.

Arrive at court in plenty of time and then be prepared to wait. If those in control of the case have specified a particular time then be available immediately outside the courtroom at that time, but still be prepared to wait. Courts are notorious for not running to time, this results from the vagaries of the adversarial system and of people. It cannot be helped and it does not result from any personal animosity towards the healthcare professional. It has to be tolerated. When you do arrive identify yourself to the court usher at the earliest opportunity. To the old adage for giving evidence in court of 'Stand up, Speak up and Shut up' can be added Dress up.

Wear smart clothes appropriate for your gender. Though the sartorial presentation has no effect on the quality of your mind and ability to give evidence, the overall impression of professionalism is important for those assessing the evidence. It is becoming more common that witnesses are invited to sit while giving evidence. If you chose to sit do not slouch, it looks bad and also impedes voice projection. Many of those who give evidence frequently still prefer to stand, consider doing so.

Speak clearly and slowly. The judge or magistrate will be making notes. In a criminal trial the jury is invariably on the other side of the room and the one at the back needs to hear the evidence.

Answer the questions put to you honestly and fully. Generally do not offer information for which you have not been asked. However if you feel you have evidence which you believe to be crucial and which has not been adduced, it is fair to indicate to the judge that you may have other material which may be relevant. This gives the opportunity for the judge to hear what you may have to say in the absence of the jury. It is possible that if you blurt out information which has already been decided is inadmissible, within the hearing of the jury, then in theory a retrial may have to be considered. That would be an expensive event which is totally avoidable. The professional witness is only usually party to a small segment of the whole case. It is the judge who has control of the running of the case and it is the judge who will decide what is admissible or not. In other words shut up.

Once in the witness box you will be asked to swear an oath. Prepare yourself beforehand as to which holy text you would wish to use to swear or if you would prefer to affirm. In any case indicate to the usher and the judge clearly and calmly what you wish to do. Having promised to be truthful, start your evidence and be so. In most courts the system used is an adversarial one, which means that the two opposing sides will test the evidence to get it to point in their favour. The Coroner's Court is inquisitorial. In Crown Court, for example, you will initially be asked questions by the side that called you, that is you will be examined in chief. Counsel will not, without agreement from the other advocate and leave of the judge be allowed to ask leading questions. The questions will then be somewhat circumspect. As soon as you need an aide-memoire, usually soon after, and hopefully not before, you have identified yourself and your qualifications ask if you may refer to your notes.

If the notes are contemporaneous there is never any problem in being allowed to use them. Your statement is not part of your contemporaneous notes and it is only in very strict circumstances that you will be allowed to refer to your statement, in a criminal trial. Be ready to identify any papers or texts that you may use while giving evidence. If the barrister asks to see your notes, hand them over. If they contain anything which you consider should not be disclosed, indicate to the judge that such material exists and claim Public Interest Immunity. The judge will then decide what is disclosable or not and to whom it may be disclosed. Otherwise just hand them over. Consent for disclosure should have been obtained during the original examination or when a report was requested.

After the examination in chief, you will be cross-examined by the opposing barrister. Here you may be asked leading questions. It has sometimes been said the cross-examination is an examination that makes you cross. Do not get cross. There are a number of good rules when being cross-examined,

1 do not get cross
2 do not behave arrogantly, justice may suffer
3 do not try to play the comic
4 do not try to play word games with the advocates, they are trained for it, and in control of the agenda, you will lose
5 do answer questions as simply as accuracy will allow
6 do concede if a concession is correct, this will make those areas on which you should not be conceding all the more potent
7 do not answer complex questions with a 'yes' or a 'no' if that is misleading

  8 if asked a complex or multiple question, break it down into its component parts and indicate that you will answer each part separately, then do so

  9 if asked a really convoluted question or any question which you do not understand ask the advocate to repeat it

10 do not get drawn out of your area of competence

12 if you do not know the answer to a question say so, you will be all the more respected for doing so

13 if shown another document or reference ask for time to read it properly it would be extremely unlikely that any judge would not allow you such time.

After the cross-examination you may be re-examined by the first counsel, who will confine any questions to material already covered.

Occasionally there are multi-handed trials with more than one defendant, in such cases there will be a barrister for each defendant, and you may be subject to more than one encounter of cross-examination, be prepared for it. Similarly in child cases there may be a counsel representing the child as well as prosecution and defence barristers so you may get multiple tiers of questioning.

Sometimes the judge will ask a question on his/her own behalf or on behalf of the jury. Again answer clearly and concisely. When giving evidence, pace steadily what you say. Make sure you are clear in your own mind what you wish to say. When you have finished giving evidence, if no one else asks on the judge on your behalf, ask if you can be released. Until you are released you should not leave the court premises. On leaving say 'thank you', you may feel no gratitude but it is polite to so do.

Use lay language, and if you have to use a technical term explain it in lay terms. Do remember you are not there to represent any side. You may feel sorry for the complainant for instance, but it is the court which will decide the guilt or innocence of the defendant. If you give evidence fairly and honestly the court is in a better position to judge the issues. If you are not objective you are objectionable.

In inquisitorial systems, such as a Coroner's Court, you may only face questions from the person presiding over the court, though rights of audience you may face questioning from advocates representing specific interests in the case, family members or other interested persons.

Index